D0612654

The Chromium Connection

A Lesson in Nutrition

by Betty Kamen, Ph.D.

Nutrition Encounter, Novato, CA 94948

All of the facts in this book have been very carefully researched, and have been drawn from the scientific literature. In no way, however, are any of the suggestions meant to take the place of advice given by physicians. Please consult a medical or health professional should the need for one be indicated.

First printing: 1990
Second printing: 1992
Third printing: 1994

Nutrition Encounter, Inc., 1990
PO Box 5847
Novato, CA 94948-5847

Printed in the United States of America
ISBN 0-944501-08-7

Dedicated to:

Walter Mertz, M.D.

Director of the Human Nutrition Research Center
of the
United States Department of Agriculture
who,
through brilliant research,
discovered
GTF chromium, and in so doing
contributed the ultimate gift to humankind:
Dr. Mertz raised
the hopes and health
of untold people the world over

Betty Kamen is an award-winning photojournalist, with graduate degrees in psychology and nutrition education. She is a nationally-known lecturer, radio/TV host, and author of many major books, hundreds of articles, and several tapes on health and nutrition. For many years, she hosted *Nutrition 57* on WMCA in New York, followed by *Nutrition Watch* on KNBR in San Francisco.

Other Books by Betty Kamen, Ph.D.

Total Nutrition During Pregnancy:
How To Be Sure You and Your Baby
Are Eating the Right Stuff

Total Nutrition for the Breast-Feeding Mother

Kids Are What They Eat:
What Every Parent Needs to Know About Nutrition

In Pursuit of Youth: Everyday Nutrition

Osteoporosis:
What It Is, How to Prevent It, How to Stop It

Nutrition In Nursing: The New Approach
A Handbook of Nursing Science

Sesame: The Superfood Seed
How It Can Add Vitality To Your Life

Siberian Ginseng:
Up-To-Date Research on the Fabled Tonic Herb

Germanium: A New Approach to Immunity

Startling New Facts About Osteoporosis:
Why Calcium Alone Does Not Prevent Bone Disease

New Facts About Fiber

Everything You Always Wanted to Know About Potassium
But Were Too Tired to Ask

Hormone Replacement Therapy: Yes or No?
How to Make an Informed Decision

CONTENTS

ACKNOWLEDGMENTS

Michael Rosenbaum, M.D., for being a select and caring member of the medical profession.

Gary Price Todd, M.D., for pioneering work correlating chromium deficiencies with diabetes and serious eye disorders.

Serafina Corsello, M.D., for friendship and the offering of unique awareness of science truths.

Richard Anderson, Ph.D., for contributions that have helped to clarify the complexities of chromium metabolism.

Dan Nidess, for providing the vehicle through which books like this get into the hands of people who benefit from them.

Paul Kamen, for patience and help offered to those of us who suffer from high-tech illiteracy.

Perle Kinney, for being there, whenever and however needed.

Joanne Catz, Professor Bernice Goldmark, Diana Dalton, and Diana Hanssen for refining judgment, clarifying language and challenging concepts.

FOREWORD

Glucose tolerance factor. Anabolic. Carbohydrate-loading. Complex carbohydrates. A few years ago, these terms were the exclusive province of the medical world. Although not exactly household words at the present time, they are appearing in media print more frequently.

In this book, Betty Kamen explains how and why chromium is the common denominator for all these "new" biological buzzwords. She recounts the history of the nutritional importance of trace quantities of chromium, established as being an essential mineral in 1959. This discovery, made by Dr. Walter Mertz of the United States Department of Agriculture, has been hailed as having one of the most significant and far-reaching effects on the nutritional aspects of human disease in the mid-twentieth century. But until Betty's compilation of the research, information about this crucial nutrient has been a "sleeper."

Chromium, found in required amounts in most young children, is not detected at all in 15 to 23 percent of Americans over the age of fifty. Yet 98.5 percent of most foreign people in that age category can boast its presence in sufficient amounts. As for the rest of our population, short supplies subject almost every one of us to many problems, both subtle and serious.

New studies consistently add to the evidence that human chromium deficiency is a formidable challenge. Chromium depletion is one etiologic factor that has to be considered in a variety of disorders. Disturbed glucose metabolism and decreased energy caused by chromium deficiency is rampant.

Increased mortality and decreased longevity are among the more critical consequences. Betty Kamen has explicitly defined the problem and the potential solutions.

You will learn that chromium functions in a special niacin-bound organic complex called *glucose tolerance factor* (GTF), which regulates carbohydrate, fat, and protein metabolism in the production of energy and in muscle development. Inorganic chromium is poorly absorbed and has only limited biological activity. GTF chromium enhances *insulin*, one of your body's most powerful anabolic hormones.

Betty explains that you are unquestionably dependent on a dietary source of GTF chromium for many aspects of good health. This is really a book about nutrition and how to attain more energy, better athletic performance, more stable blood sugar metabolism, weight loss, cholesterol and heart health, and better stress-coping abilities. Just about everyone—lay people and professionals—will find this book remarkably helpful.

Michael E. Rosenbaum, M.D.
45 San Clemente Drive
Corte Madera, CA 94941
(415) 927-9450

AUTHOR'S NOTE

I am in awe of the myriad cells in the human body. Some of these endless cells work alone and some take charge of others through a complex system of chemical signals, existing in dense interdependent communities. Most cells collaborate and accomodate. Yet each, regardless of function, is a microcosm all by itself—with an internal hustle and bustle that makes the pace of New York City restrained by comparison.

Our food supply has detached itself from nature. This external influence has been overpowering our internal machinery, interfering with the way our cells send messages to each other, disturbing their designated work.

The great scientists of the world are helping us emerge from this dilemma. One in particular has been doing research in the area of *blood sugar metabolism*, a process influenced by our environment to such a degree that many people suffer in many different ways.

In the late 1950s, Dr. Walter Mertz, a United States government researcher, made an important discovery. He found that animals fed chromium-deficient Torula yeast developed diabetic-like symptoms. But when chromium-rich brewer's yeast was administered, the symptoms disappeared. Dr. Mertz' discovery led to the identification of the *glucose tolerance factor,* or GTF, as it has come to be known. GTF is an organic chromium complex that binds insulin to cell membrane receptor sites. At these receptor sites, insulin tranports blood sugar (glucose) and vital amino acids inside cells for energy and protein synthesis.

Although Dr. Mertz was unable to decipher the exact molecular structure of GTF, he determined that the essential component of the complex was the *chromium-niacin* axis.

To prove this, Dr. Mertz performed experiments to measure insulin sensitivity in the presence of both niacin-bound chromium and chromium bound to niacin *isomers.* (Niacin isomers are chemical compounds that are nearly identical to niacin.) He then compared the insulin-activating effects of these compounds with pure GTF extracted from brewer's yeast. The chromium-niacin complex activated insulin equally as well as pure GTF, but the chromium-isomer compounds proved to be ineffective.

Even though the molecules of the isomers are almost identical to the molecules of niacin, *almost identical* just doesn't work in nature. *Almost identical* is the structure of the DNA molecule of humans and apes, or the DNA that separates a normal child from one with Downs Syndrome—to cite just a few examples.

As a result of recent research, we now have considerable insight into the mechanisms of the glucose tolerance factor, and also the development of interesting new supplements. A major university study shows that the chromium-niacin compound, *chromium polynicotinate*, significantly lowers cholesterol.

Other research has proved that niacin-bound chromium supplementation is helpful in several additional areas. You may want to ask your physician about the use of chromium polynicotinate supplementation if you:

- cannot lose weight
- want to have more energy
- are under stress
- overreact to ordinary circumstances

- participate in any form of athletics or aerobics
- have any problems with blood sugar metabolism
- sustain elevated cholesterol levels
- suffer from heart disease
- just want to insure your good health

Yes, the environment, which has decreased vital chromium supplies, has affected those cells which impact on all the processes listed. As your cells communicate, some of the messages they send to each other have become distorted because the trace mineral chromium, needed for their proper function, is missing! This book explains how you can overcome these problems.

It is with great enthusiasm that I write about chromium polynicotinate. As an antidote for weight gain and low-blood-sugar reactions, this supplement has more than fulfilled its promise for me personally.

The need for energy is quantitatively the largest single nutritive factor (with the exception of water). Although other food factors are important, their shortages are not as significantly apparent. *Chromium polynicotinate can help to maximize energy potential.*

Betty Kamen, Ph.D.

ADDENDUM: *Second Printing*

Medical literature continues to validate the information presented in this book. Note the following:

»**Chromium polynicotinate**. A new (as yet unpublished) study shows that niacin-bound chromium polynicotinate is absorbed significantly faster and better than chromium chloride or chromium picolinate. Researchers used radio-active isotopes of the chromium compounds being studied to measure the absorption, retention, and excretion rates. These tests were done in seven different tissue groups on laboratory animals.

»**Insulin, diabetes, low blood sugar.** In the presence of optimal amounts of biologically active chromium, much lower amounts of insulin are required. Glucose intolerance, related to insufficient dietary chromium, appears to be widespread. Improved chromium nutrition leads to improved sugar metabolism in hypoglycemics, hyperglycemics, and diabetics.
Biological Trace Element Research, 1992

»**Triglycerides, cholesterol**. Seventy-six patients with atherosclerotic disease were treated daily with either 250 micrograms of chromium orally or a placebo for a period of 7 to 16 months. Triglycerides were lower and high-density lipoprotein increased in the patients who received the chromium.
Metabolism, 1992.

»**Need for chromium supplementation well established**. Trivalent chromium lowers blood levels of low density lipoproteins (LDL), raises high density lipoproteins (HDL) and improves glucose tolerance. Chromium deficiency can be established by the reversal of symptoms and signs following the administration of trivalent chromium. This evidence can be

supported by knowledge or suspicion of a deficiency in the diet, *common in those who use highly refined* cereal foods. It is considered that the beneficial effects of chromium repletion are now so well established and the trivalent form is so free of toxicity that it should now be used in clinical medicine for the benefit of those with some forms of diabetes and its complications and those suffering from atherosclerosis.
Central African Journal of Medicine, 1991.

»**Exercise**. Because of the low intakes of chromium for the general population, there is a possibility that athletes may be deficient. Exercise may create a loss in chromium because of increased excretion into the urine. Poor diets are perhaps the main reason for any mineral deficiencies found in athletes, although in certain cases exercise could contribute to the deficiency. Mineral supplementation may be important to ensure good health.
Journal of Sports Sciences, 1991.

»**Cereal refinement**. Chromium is discarded in the cereal refinement process. We now have added evidence for a return to the diets in which complex carbohydrates predominated. In those who refuse or are unable to do this, the addition of chromium may be of value.
Central African Journal of Medicine, 1991.

»**Men on beta-blockers.** Two months of chromium supplementation resulted in a clinically useful increase in HDL cholesterol levels in men taking beta-blockers.
Annals of Internal Medicine, 1991

These are just a few of the current studies.

BK

ADDENDUM: *Third Printing*

When this book was first printed in 1990, it was ahead of its time. Chromium has now come into its own: it is finally recognized as one of the most important nutrients. Both traditional and alternative practitioners recommend supplemental chromium. As we go into our third printing, even more studies support the conclusions cited.

The nutrition department of the University of California at Davis found chromium polynicotinate (ChromeMate) to be absorbed several hundredfold better than other forms of chromium.

The United States Department of Agriculture found that the amount of chromium nicotinate retained in tissue is also significantly higher than that retained with other forms.

A study at Auburn University showed that niacin-bound chromium lowered cholesterol an average of 14 percent and improved total cholesterol/HDL ratios by 7 percent.

These results reinforce the 20 years of research that began with Dr. Mertz's discovery of the chromium-niacin axis in brewer's yeast. Niacin is an essential B-vitamin for humans and is acknowledged as the ligand for chromium in biologically active chromium.

CHAPTER 1

CHROMIUM

what it is, what it does, where it is found

GLOSSARY

adaptogen - substance normalizing functions indirectly.

bioavailability - the degree to which a substance becomes available to a target tissue after administration.

biological activity - processes connected with living matter.

blood sugar - glucose circulating in blood; principal fuel for most body cells (see *glucose* below).

brewer's yeast - by-product left after brewing; contains high amount of chromium.

cataract - cloudiness in lens of eye, reducing amount of light going through.

chromium - trace metal required in minute amounts for metabolism of blood sugar and efficiency of many other functions.

chromium/niacin complex - principal precursor of biological GTF activity.

insulin receptor sites - molecules located on outer surface and internal membranes of cells which bind insulin to facilitate the transport of glucose across membranes.

glucose - chief product of carbohydrate digestion; simple sugar present in blood and other tissues; serves as major source of immediate fuel for cells.

GTF chromium - glucose tolerance factor; organic chromium complex responsible for binding insulin to cell membrane receptor sites; active component in brewer's yeast.

lipids - fats; used with reference to biochemistry of fats—whereas the word "fat" is usually applied in connection with food content and tissues; the two words are more or less interchangeable.

metabolism - collective name for all physical and chemical changes taking place in living organisms affecting vital processes of cells.

niacin - member of vitamin B-complex; also referred to as B_3.

precursor - substance necessary for the manufacture of another substance; the source of another substance.

trace mineral - element required in very small amounts.

CHROMIUM AS AN ADAPTOGEN

Accelerated aging processes may be average, but they are not necessarily normal.

CHROMIUM: WHAT IT IS

ESSENTIAL TRACE MINERALS

Hard to imagine, isn't it? Some essential trace elements occupy no more—and usually many times less—than 0.01 percent of your body. Yet this barely perceptible quantity is critical to your health! In fact, the impact of these elements is so profound that serious abnormalities may result even if you are slightly deficient in any one of them.

To date, sixteen such metals have been identified as necessary for human nutrition. Coined as *essential trace elements*, you must eat these nutrients because your body cannot produce them in adequate amounts, if at all.

Some have been referred to as *ultratrace* because they are found in extremely minute proportions.

The seventeenth century gave us iron—the first essential trace element to be identified. During the Middle Ages, iron nails were inserted in apples and allowed to rust to produce an iron supplement for children. Centuries earlier, the Greeks had recognized the importance of iron. An ancient story reveals that Melampus, ship's surgeon to Jason and the

Argonauts, supplemented wine with filings from iron swords to help counter blood loss and amplify sexual potency.

The most recently recognized in this limited group of essential trace elements is cadmium, uncovered as a necessary mineral for humans in 1976. Reports of the dangers of cadmium toxicity from the environment have been overwhelming through the years, but we now know that cadmium-deficient diets are also a possibility, and are related to poor growth and other problems.[1]

Because today's high technology allows us to calculate almost everything with great specificity, it has been proposed that the term *essential trace elements* be abandoned, and that *all* elements be regarded as "essential biological metals."[2] Meanwhile, the designation *trace element* continues to be used.

Elements, in general, attest to a certain uniformity in nature: those found in large proportions in humans are plentiful in both plants and animals; those discovered in mere traces in humans are found only in marginal amounts in plants and animals.

A trace element, however, is more than a necessary substance existing in meager quantities. Here are additional criteria:

»A trace element must be present in all healthy tissues of all living beings, although quantities may vary considerably in different tissues. (Chromium, for example, differs as much as ten-fold from one organ of your body to another.)

»When withdrawn from *any* species, a trace element induces the *same* aberrations.

»The addition of the trace element either prevents or reverses these abnormalities.[3]

»A trace element may be toxic when given in very high amounts, but not in intermediate doses.

»Health-related advantages of trace elements are best demonstrated when a deficiency state exists; when the element is administered, we can see how much depends on it.[4]

CHROMIUM IS A TYPICAL EXAMPLE OF AN ESSENTIAL TRACE MINERAL.

ADAPTOGENS

Substances which help to normalize body functions indirectly are known as *adaptogens.* A true adaptogen has little influence on healthy functions, but significantly and favorably affects responses which are out of alignment. Because of this capability, *an adaptogen may help to prevent degenerative disease and assist in slowing down the aging process.*

When adaptogens are supplied to healthy young animals, little advantage is achieved. But don't dismiss adaptogens on this basis. Healthy test animals are not difficult to breed. In today's polluted and plastic world, not many humans enjoy optimal health at *any* age. That's why *almost every human can benefit from adaptogens.*

Adaptogens are usually nutritional in origin and differ from drugs in several ways:

»No prescriptions are necessary. Adaptogens answer the need for those who say, "What can I do at home so that I won't have to go to the doctor?" Or, "What can I do to reduce the deleterious effects of the drug treatment prescribed by my physician?"

»Adaptogens are user-friendly. No professional expertise, high-tech equipment, needles, or syringes are required for administration when taken in recommended quantities.

»Adaptogens cost less than most drugs.

»Adaptogens are not habit forming.

»A drug continues to work even after a state of normalcy is achieved. Adaptogens regulate, and are held in abeyance when the challenge ceases to exist.

GTF CHROMIUM AS AN ADAPTOGEN

Here's an example of an adaptogenic paradigm: A study reported in the *American Journal of Clinical Nutrition* demonstrated that malnourished children in Turkey, Jordan, and Nigeria consumed diets low in chromium. The children responded to supplemental chromium with improvements in glucose tolerance (blood sugar management). But malnourished children in Egypt who consumed a diet *high* in chromium did not respond to the supplemental therapy.[5]

An organic chromium complex called *GTF chromium* is an *adaptogen*. (GTF stands for *glucose tolerance factor*.) It helps to normalize chromium-dependent functions only if chromium is in short supply.

You will learn that *GTF chromium encourages a response that depends on your degree of need.*[6] This same concept applies to so many familiar natural substances.

Let's set the record straight about chromium: we are not talking about making your insides beaming, bright, or brilliant, the role of commercial chrome plating. The type of chromium that is an artifact of industrial processing—known as *hexavalent* chromium—is very different from the chromium found in nature, and is highly toxic. Natural, or biological, chromium is *trivalent*, and is the more abundant of the two forms. (The valence of a substance is a measure of the capacity of that substance to combine with other elements. Hexavalent, Cr^{+6}, has six bonding points; trivalent, Cr^{+3}, has three.)

CHROMIUM: WHAT IT DOES

CHROMIUM IS MULTIFACETED

It is only natural that we are skeptical when we hear about a long list of spectacular benefits associated with a single substance. Any drug or nutrient—or even a food—said to be in control of more than one aspect of health is difficult to comprehend. In our culture, we usually regard such substances as snake oil and its messenger a quack. This view stems from the allopathic specialization of American medicine. The allopathic approach often assumes that illness, or abnormal function, has a solitary cause and effect, unrelated to any other disease state. Therefore, a specific disease is treated with a single agent, targeted only for the disorder at hand. For example, I was taught that vitamin A was good for my eyes; that calcium was needed for my bones. And that was that. New waves are washing away these old descriptive liaisons. Medicine is no longer considered a narrow, organ-based pathological system. Current thinking supports the view that disease or health is part of a spectrum, with much wider boundaries than previously theorized.

Vitamin A *is* good for your vision, and calcium *is* required for bone health, but these facts are only the tip of the iceberg. Each of these nutrients plays an important role in myriad *other* functions; yet, neither nutrient can perform its designated job alone. A single note of music cannot create a melody. Today's biochemistry unites studies at both cellular and whole-animal levels, insight brought about by unprecedented scientific thinking and modern technology.

THE DISTINCTIONS OF CHROMIUM

The change in medical perception described above led to the recognition of the importance of chromium and helps to explain *why* and *how* one trace element can be involved in so many diverse reactions. In addition to the processes listed in the chart below, chromium impacts on your immune system, and—are you paying attention?—*it helps to delay the aging process! Accelerated aging processes may be average, but they are not necessarily normal.*

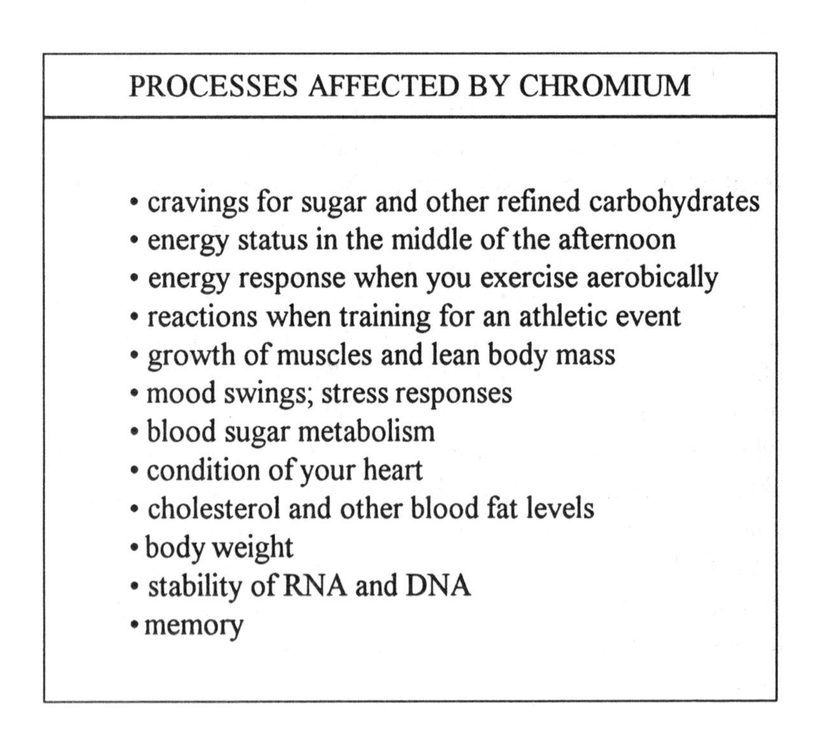

PROCESSES AFFECTED BY CHROMIUM

- cravings for sugar and other refined carbohydrates
- energy status in the middle of the afternoon
- energy response when you exercise aerobically
- reactions when training for an athletic event
- growth of muscles and lean body mass
- mood swings; stress responses
- blood sugar metabolism
- condition of your heart
- cholesterol and other blood fat levels
- body weight
- stability of RNA and DNA
- memory

All this and heaven too, since you only require an infinitesimal amount of chromium to accomplish these vital life functions, and (we are told) trace elements are present in many foods. So we must be getting more than enough. Right? Not so. Read on.

HISTORY: THE BREAKTHROUGH

Although discovered two hundred years ago, chromium was not identified as essential for humans until 1959. Prior to that, scientists were able to use chromium to stimulate or inhibit enzyme systems in a test tube, as reported in prestigious journals of biology and biochemistry.[7,8] Researchers knew something important was happening, but the details were vague. Because chromium is active at such low levels, it was difficult to induce chromium deficiency in laboratory animals.

The breakthrough came when Dr. Walter Mertz, while at the National Institute of Health in Bethesda, Maryland, observed that feeding a chromium-deficient diet to test animals resulted in severe impairment of their ability to metabolize *glucose*. Since part of everything you eat turns into this simple sugar, the discovery was momentous.

The recognition of the importance of chromium led to the discovery of the *glucose tolerance factor* (GTF), an organic chromium complex responsible for binding insulin to cell-membrane receptor sites. (In later chapters, you will learn what this means and why it is so important.) Trivalent chromium is the center of this compound, and niacin molecules and a few amino acids are also present. Dr. Mertz identified this niacin/chromium complex as part of the active component in brewer's yeast.[9] The amino acids are believed to help with transportation—moving the nutrient complex through your system.

GTF CHROMIUM: DEFINING THE REAL THING

Noting the differences between GTF and simple chromium, Dr. Mertz set standards by which GTF chromium could be distinguished from the inactive variety. He explained the reasons for setting these standards. Since the exact structure of GTF is not known, GTF chromium should be identified by characteristics based on what it *does*, rather than on what it *is*; that is, on *biological activity* rather than on *chemical structure*. (Biological activity is that fraction of the element in a food that is absorbed and utilized.[10]) Like so many other phenomena in advanced science, we benefit from limited knowledge. If we waited for a full understanding of electricity, we'd still be sitting in the dark. The same applies to gravity and space travel.

STANDARDS FOR IDENTIFYING GTF CHROMIUM
• helps glucose enter cells because of its action on insulin • is absorbed better than simple chromium compounds • has access to special tissue stores within the body • crosses the placenta and incorporates into the fetus • is significantly less toxic than simple chromium compounds

Other researchers subsequently concurred with Dr. Mertz. *The general concensus is that chromium is well-absorbed when given orally in the trivalent form in a particular infra-structure; absorption is also affected by the functional state of your intestine; it is able to cross the placenta as a specific natural complex, but not as a simple salt; and the margin between essentiality and toxicity is substantial, so that large doses are safe.*

CHROMIUM FINDINGS: PAST AND PRESENT

Sir William Osler, doctor-hero of the medical profession, cautioned physicians against the arrogance of believing that only current medical practices can benefit a patient. If new information is spread effectively, everyone becomes better educated, and we begin to narrow the gap between the pace of research and the application of new knowledge.

Researchers and clinicians uncovered a huge mass of brand-new information since the early days of Dr. Mertz' initial chromium explorations (which are still ongoing). Here are pertinent findings, both recent and past.

»GTF chromium is a hormone-like compound. One of its main functions is to regulate sugar metabolism. Even if refined sugar is totally absent from your diet, chromium is necessary because foods are eventually reduced to simple glucose, your body's primary source of energy.

»Nucleic acids contain very high concentrations of chromium. The *Journal of Biology and Chemistry* and *Physiology Review* report that chromium is important for the metabolism, structure, and integrity of the nuclear strands.[11,12] Nucleic acids are found in the nucleus of all living cells and are essential to life. They are the carriers of genetic information.

»The highest amounts of chromium occur at birth, decreasing as you get older.

FOR MALES, THE TESTES ARE THE ORGAN MOST AFFECTED BY AGING CHROMIUM REDUCTION.[13]

A large survey on the distribution of trace metals in the human body was reported in a book on metals in medicine. The survey shows that chromium is unique in its decline with increasing age. This study, conducted thirty years ago, concluded that chromium is the *only* trace mineral diminishing with age.[14] A more accurate statement would probably be: *Chromium loss as you age is more extensive than that of any other trace element.*

»The quantity of chromium in specific table foods cannot be easily measured. The limited amounts that are present vary with the supply in the soil, and with the degree of food refinement.

Another reason why chromium in food cannot be measured easily is that differences in bioavailability exist between GTF and inorganic chromium.[15] (Bioavailability refers to a substance that is biologically accessible for use by the tissue for which it is intended.) Leaching of inorganic chromium from stainless steel pots and blender blades into foods and beverages is well-documented.[16,17] Inorganic chromium shows up in analyses, but your body cannot always convert inorganic chromium to its useful form. Such transformation is dependent on the presence of synergistic nutrients—*other nutrients necessary for the conversion to take place*. And your capability of making the changeover declines as you get older.

»Dr. Henry Schroeder, in *The Trace Elements and Man,* describes how chromium helps to mitigate the harmful effects of certain toxic substances. When chromium-deficient test animals are given an excess of lead, mortality due to infection occurs. When the lead-exposed animals are given chromium supplements, no such death takes place.[18] Decreased blood chromium levels are associated with acute infectious disease, as confirmed in reports given in *Federal Proceedings.*[19]

For this reason, it has been suggested that taking additional supplements of chromium at the start of a cold might help to nip your respiratory infection in the bud.

»The need for chromium is greater under certain circumstances.

CIRCUMSTANCES INCREASING CHROMIUM NEEDS
• athletic and aerobic involvement • impaired glucose metabolism a) diabetes b) low blood sugar • pregnancy • lactation • atherosclerotic heart disease • low birthweight

»Less insulin is required when levels of chromium are high. Although chromium potentiates the action of insulin, it does not replace it. In the same way, a more efficient engine uses less gas, but its efficiency doesn't substitute for gas. You get "more miles per gallon" with active forms of chromium. Insulin function is optimized.

»Glucose is a vital source of energy for normal growth and development of the fetus. Because high levels of glucose are required for transportation across the placenta, chromium doesn't remain a maternal passenger for long. This information was highlighted in an international newsletter I receive from Hyderabad.[20] Since chromium can only cross the placenta in its GTF form, it has been considered a "vitamin" for the fetus. *The American Journal of Obstetrics and Gynecology* confirms that an optimal supply is dependent on an adequate dietary source for the mother.

BY THE TIME THE AVERAGE AMERICAN WOMAN REACHES HER THIRD TRIMESTER, HER CHROMIUM LEVELS ARE LOWER THAN THOSE OF NONPREGNANT WOMEN.[21]

Undoubtedly related, premature infants rarely have enough chromium.[22]

»Another site of chromium action is your eye. Test animals ingesting low chromium diets and diets high in protein develop an opaque cornea and congestion of the iris.[23]

»Chromium has been used successfully for the treatment of cataracts, and for macular degeneration. Gary Price Todd, M.D., of Waynesville, North Carolina, has been able to completely reverse cataracts in early stages.[24]

»The National Research Council placed chromium on the charts in 1977, recommending from 50 to 200 micrograms a day as a safe and adequate range. (A microgram is one-thousandth of a milligram; a milligram is one-thousandth of a gram; 28 grams equals an ounce. Or, a microgram is one-billionth of a kilogram, which is 2.2 pounds.)

»When small amounts of chromium are added to the diet, vitamin C metabolism increases.[25] Because vitamin C is such a fragile nutrient, easily destroyed by cooking and processing, any potentiation of its use is beneficial.

»Just how chromium is absorbed is unknown. Absorption appears to be dependent on body stores, dietary intake, and on the bioavailability of the form consumed. Unlike other trace elements, chromium doesn't function as a pure metal. It appears to require the formation of a highly specialized organic complex, which includes niacin, the B vitamin. Dr. Mertz demonstrated that niacin-bound GTF chromium increases bioavailability.[26]

»Chromium absorption also depends on other foods eaten during the same meal.

OXALATES INCREASE CHROMIUM ABSORPTION
PHYTATES DECREASE CHROMIUM ABSORPTION

Oxalate Foods	Phytate Foods
• spinach	• cheese
• unhulled sesame	• other dairy products
• beet greens	• soft drinks
• parsley	• processed foods

»New studies confirm that sugar produces a major impairment of insulin action by adversely affecting chromium absorption.[27] It's a tug of war: foods generally regarded as healthful improve chromium status, just as those that are not will erode it.

»Studies show that chromium bolsters protein manufacture in your liver.[28]

»Dr. Richard Anderson writes in *Metabolism* that chromium deficiency can be invoked by coronary heart disease, exercise, injury, illness, and other forms of stress.[29] It is often present in the offspring of diabetic mothers.

»Once chromium deficiency is under way, for whatever reason, it can cause a long list of disease states and symptoms, including diabetes, hypoglycemia, atherosclerosis, fatigue, weight problems, retarded growth, plaques in large blood vessels, corneal lesions, shortened lifespan, lower sperm count, high cholesterol levels, and lipid metabolism problems. And that's not all! The list goes on and on.

»The effects of marginal chromium deficiency are slow to develop. It may take several years before overt signs of deficiency surface enough to be measured.[30] Common signs of marginal chromium deficiency which are alleviated by increased dietary intake of chromium include impaired glucose tolerance, elevated circulating insulin, decreased insulin binding and receptor number, elevated cholesterol and triglycerides, and decreased high density lipoprotein cholesterol.[31,32]

EITHER AS CAUSE OR EFFECT,
RHEUMATOID ARTHRITICS HAVE
VERY LOW LEVELS OF CHROMIUM,
AS REPORTED IN THE
JOURNAL OF CHRONIC DISEASES.[33]

»When fed chromium-deficient diets, the pancreas of a test animal becomes enlarged, indicating that chromium deficiency alters pancreatic function.[34]

»Blood chromium drops precipitously when glucose is given intravenously. If a postoperative patient also has a viral infection, blood chromium can drop even more. The end result may be disastrous. The addition of GTF chromium has been recommended for patients requiring glucose solutions.

»Compared with normal subjects, the average amount of chromium in the livers of those who die of hypertension, arteriosclerosis, and diabetes is significantly lower. Hypertensives have about 18 percent less chromium; arteriosclerotics 25 percent less; diabetics 33 percent less.[35]

YOUR LIFE QUALITY HAS THE POTENTIAL TO BE IMPAIRED IF YOU LACK THIS MINUSCULE AMOUNT OF CHROMIUM.

Impressive and yet scary, isn't it? But no matter your age, your health can improve greatly. At no point in life is anyone so bound to an ill state that at least some measure of change for the better cannot be initiated when given the tools with which to work.

CHROMIUM: WHERE IT IS FOUND

AMERICANS AND CHROMIUM DEFICIENCY

Because chromium has been shown to be an essential element in fungi and in vertebrates, anthropologists tell us that it has been present in air and water throughout the evolution of plants and animals.[36] Today, traces of chromium can be detected in air sampled at sites remote from human life. Analysis of these samples indicates that some of the airborne chromium comes from wind-blown soil.[37]

It may not surprise you, then, that humans have lower chromium than levels measured in wild animals. What is shocking is that if you lived in almost any other country but the United States, you would have more chromium in your cells. According to the United States Department of Agriculture, *suboptimal chromium is common in our country*. Among Americans over fifty, as many as 25 percent may have negligible chromium levels, and 90 percent of those eating an average American diet receive less than the government's recommended daily allowance, little as that is. A seven-day average chromium intake was observed among normal, affluent Americans. This group claimed to have better-than-average knowledge of good nutritional practices. It was proved that *none consumed the minimum suggested amount of chromium.*[38,39]

WHY WE ARE DEFICIENT

Plant foods tend to be a poor source of chromium due to the low content in our agricultural soil. When chromium is present, it occurs in a form poorly translocated from the root of a plant to its stems or leaves. Intentional efforts to increase the chromium content in edible seed crops have failed.

None of the plants normally used as animal feed or for human consumption accumulates chromium. It is one of the few essential elements that does not accrue at any stage in the biological cycle from soil to plant to animal.[40]

Baked products such as crackers, pastries, bread, and pasta made with white flour are chromium-deficient. Eighty percent or more of the chromium has been removed as a result of milling—the process converting whole grains to refined flours.[41] Commercial treatment of foods in preparation for canning or freezing (trimming, leaching, blanching, adding preservatives, or heating), contributes to significant additional losses. Dr. Stephen Tannenbaum, in *Principles of Food Science*, warns that *all processed foods are subject to some degree of mineral content casualties.*[42]

Chromium was tallied in diets designed by registered dietitians. One-third contained less than 50 micrograms daily. *Even the professionals have difficulty getting enough chromium from the food supply!*[43]

FORMULA:
SUGAR IN = CHROMIUM OUT

When the effects of aerobic exercise and training on chromium were tested, *Sports Medicine* reported that refined sugar is the one single substance that causes the greatest chromium excretion.[44] Consuming chocolate, ketchup, sweet desserts, most cold breakfast cereals, cola and other soft drinks, or any other foods high in simple sugars, causes you to increase chromium losses up to 300 percent. The higher the percentage of sugar in your diet, the greater the chromium losses.[45,46]

SUGAR IS DOUBLE-TROUBLE BECAUSE IT LACKS CHROMIUM TO BEGIN WITH, AND THEN STIMULATES MORE CHROMIUM LOSS.

It is no wonder that when Dr. Todd tested 800 patients he found that 96 percent were chromium deficient.[47] And no wonder that my children, like George Bush, complained about nutrients being in the broccoli instead of in the ice cream.

CHROMIUM LOSSES CAUSED BY FOOD PROCESSING	
• White flour	98 percent loss
• Sugar refining	95 percent loss
• Rice polishing	92 percent loss
• Corn starch	100 percent loss
• Skimmed or fat-free milk	100 percent loss
• Cooking (at home or at canning factory)	Additional losses
• Vegetable peeling (as in freezing processes)	Additional losses

Refined and fractionated foods are indicted as the principal causes for the following differences in chromium content:[48,49,50]

- 2.00 parts per billion (ppb) in sea water
- 0.60 ppb in primitive man
- 0.09 ppb in modern man

CHROMIUM ANTAGONISTS

The lack of chromium in food is not the only reason for chromium deficiencies. An extensive roster of chromium adversaries—factors which are antagonistic to chromium—add to the problem.

CHROMIUM DESTROYERS

- air pollution
- emotional stress
- physical stress: heat, cold, or exercise
- radiation
- change in hormonal balance (diabetes and low blood sugar head the list)
- acute infectious states: colds, etc.
- repeated pregnancies
- age
- excessive iron and/or zinc in diet
- excessive vanadium (found in kelp and large fish)

You now have an idea why we have chromium levels two to three times lower than those in primitive societies.[51]

CHROMIUM IN FOOD

The best known source of chromium is brewer's yeast. Chromium also occurs in significant amounts in mammalian liver and kidney tissues, and in the bran and germ portions of cereal grains (with the exception of corn and rye). Chromium is present, but to a lesser degree, in molasses, the skin of apples, beer, prunes, American cheese, some shell fish, mushrooms, wine, and black pepper. Insignificant amounts are found in most vegetables and fruit. Even water contains only small quantities. According to information given at the *Proceedings of the 12th Conference on Great Lakes Research*, the metal accrues mainly in the skin, bones, liver and kidneys of fish, parts which are normally not eaten by humans.[52]

Let's examine these "high" chromium foods.

»Brewer's yeast

An ounce of brewer's yeast contains 168 micrograms of chromium. Chances are you didn't swallow a bunch of brewer's yeast tablets today, perhaps because brewer's yeast has been maligned as an allergen, albeit mistakenly. There are more than a hundred different strains of yeast, only a few of which may cause sensitive reactions. Brewer's yeast may not be in the danger-zone for you. In fact, many clinicians report favorable accounts from patients who take supplemental brewer's yeast.

Brewer's yeast, as its name implies, is used in the preparation of beer and ale, and should not be confused with baker's yeast.

»Liver and kidneys

Three and one half ounces of liver contain 50 micrograms of chromium. What are the chances that you ate liver today? Liver is not generally a favorite food. It is also believed to be toxic, and a contributing factor for raised cholesterol. Let's dispel a few myths.

Liver is a detoxifying organ. Therefore, the antagonists say, "Toxins settle in its tissue. Don't eat it."

Liver proponents say, "Since the liver is a detoxifying organ, it gets rid of toxins. Eat it. Besides, toxins settle in fat throughout your entire body, not only in your liver."

In addition to its high chromium content, liver is a depot for *all* vitamins and minerals. Perhaps this is why native American tribes believed the human liver to be the repository of "manly" virtues.[53]

The solution is to find pesticide-free, organic sources of liver. They are available. (See Chapter 8 for a sure-to-be-liked liver recipe).

As for cholesterol content, it has never been proved that cholesterol levels are raised significantly by consuming wholesome, intact foods—even those foods with high cholesterol content. Just the opposite has been demonstrated. Hazardous cholesterol levels occur from the consumption of processed foods (especially those with transformed fats) and from stress. Many nutrition researchers have worked hard to dispel the cholesterol/heart disease fallacies. It cannot be overemphasized that natural and healthful foods containing cholesterol do *not* cause dangerous cholesterol blood levels.[34]

FOODS WITH TRANSFORMED FATS
• fried foods • salad and cooking oils • nut butters • processed baked goods • margarine and other ersatz foods • foods with hydrogenated oils

As for kidney, it is not particularly popular (unless you happen to be English and enjoy steak-and-kidney pie).

»Whole grains

Chromium is found in greatest amounts in the hulls and coarse outer portions of grains. Whole grains are usually hard to come by in convenience foods. Look carefully at the labels of supermarket whole wheat products. You will find that many contain white flour. Even if the label reads, "100 percent whole wheat," the product may be made from an impure flour lacking bran and some of the germ.[55] Whole grains do not keep as well as refined flour, nor do they have as much "hold-together" power. Refined white flour, as indicated, has lost most of its chromium.[56]

Bakers of whole grain breads and other baked goods may add gluten to recipes. Gluten, highly allergenic, is the protein fraction of wheat responsible for sensitivity reactions. It derives its name because it is sticky, giving the dough a tough elastic quality. It is, literally, the "glue" that does keep the cookie from crumbling. Although the whole wheat grain does contain some chromium, gluten contains none.[57]

That we enjoy and crave baked products and find them difficult to resist is more than a cultural phenomenon. Gluten acts as a morphine-like component. Consuming foods which contain gluten can create a drug-like euphoria. With repeated ingestion, it may become an addiction. Failure to get the "fix" causes withdrawal symptoms, which then prompts the "victim" to seek food—especially foods with gluten. And aren't most of us so victimized![58]

THE ADDICTION STARTS IN CHILDHOOD
WITH MILK AND COOKIES.
THE CASEIN IN MILK HAS ALSO BEEN
IDENTIFIED AS HAVING THE SAME
EUPHORIA-ADDICTING PATHWAY
AS GLUTEN IN WHEAT!

Needless to say, the aftermath is not as deleterious as "recreational" drugs, but you would probably be astounded at how many people suffer minor emotional and physical difficulties as a result of gluten in their diets. The natural gluten content in whole wheat is under question for many people; adding *more* gluten exacerbates the difficulty.

When I interviewed representatives from one of these bakeries, I was told they were aware of the objection, but had no choice. "Without gluten," they explained, "the baked goods would fall apart." I take exception to this excuse. There are baked products in the marketplace that do not contain added gluten. Read your labels.

So, although a cupful of whole wheat berries contains about 36 micrograms of chromium, this is hardly the amount you would be getting in processed "whole grain" products.

»Molasses

It is almost impossible to secure unadulterated, pure molasses. Because sugar beet molasses—the variety that contains high amounts of chromium—is less sweet than cane molasses, it is seldom marketed.[59] As for blackstrap molasses, it contains only 5 micrograms of chromium per tablespoon.

»Apple skin

Unless certified organic, the skin of an apple is nothing that contributes to optimal health because pesticides concentrate in the outer layers of fruit. But that's also where the nutrients are found. A tasty organic apple of medium size contains about 36 micrograms of chromium only if all the growing processes and conditions are optimal.

»Beer

Beer may be contaminated with copper from tubing used in the breweries. Malt adjuncts added to beer may be starch, sugar, or syrups. Beer may be pasteurized to prevent spoilage and also to destroy some nonheat-resistant bacteria.[60] Alcohol in general contributes to reduced bone mass.

Nutritive yeast, the healthful by-product, is extracted from beer.[61] Beer may contain chromium if it were brewed in stainless steel vats. (Stainless steel is made with chromium.) Twelve ounces of beer could contain 34 micrograms of chromium. But the negative aspects outweigh this advantage.

»Prunes

A prune is not the modest, simple food of years gone by. It is often "tenderized" by hydration, and you wind up paying fruit prices for water. Preservatives frequently used on dried fruit have unfavorable effects. (They may be coated with sulfites, which can affect asthmatics and, for that matter, *anyone* with respiratory problems.) A single prune contains about 5 micrograms of chromium, the same amount as found in a tablespoon of blackstrap molasses.

»Cheese

Most real cheese is high in fat and difficult to digest. The finished product may have been exposed to any or all of the following substances and/or processes: acid coagulators, salt, flavorings, bleaching, calcium chloride to "set" the milk in a semisolid mass, high heat, coloring to offset the yellow color of milk, mold-inhibiting ingredients for longer shelf life, antibiotics to suppress the growth of certain bacteria, wax coatings on cheese rinds, chemicals to wash the curds, and stabilizers for smooth texture and thickness.

Cheese is exceptionally high in phytates, which, as cited earlier, decrease chromium absorption. A one-inch cube of cheddar cheese contains about 9 micrograms of chromium; mozzarella cheese contains 11 micrograms.

»Shell fish

The amount of chromium varies for different species of fish. Not a bad choice, if you can find shell fish from unpolluted waters. Coastal areas, which nurture shellfish, are often contaminated with bacteria and poison-laden excrements. Fish are extremely sensitive to pesticides. They have been known to concentrate poisons two thousand-fold over the amounts in the water they swim in.

In spite of these problems, ocean fish are still among the better food selections. I eat fish, and try to counter the disadvantages with antioxidants. (And, of course, I take my niacin-bound GTF chromium.)

»Mushrooms

Mushrooms are a good complex carbohydrate, provided they are not excessively sprayed with pesticides. Mushrooms are often grown on horse manure compost. Because of the abundance of insects and bacteria, pesticides are added to the compost. Pesticide-free Reishi and shiitaki mushrooms are available at the produce sections of your health food market. One cup of raw mushrooms contains about 33 micrograms of chromium.

»Wine

Wine has its own list of adverse-reaction contributions. Alcohol is a major donator of blood lead levels, and lead concentrations in wine are higher than in any other alcoholic beverage. Lead is a calcium antagonist. (Remember that chromium is a lead antagonist! So don't rely on wine for your chromium supply, but consider taking additional chromium if you happen to be a wine drinker.)

»Black pepper

How much sprinkled black pepper could one consume? Quantities large enough to contribute to your chromium supply also contribute to high blood pressure.[62]

WHAT ABOUT EGGS?

Egg yolks, although high in chromium, contain a form of simple chromium that is normally poorly absorbed. It is possible, however, that the small amount present is better absorbed because of cofactors in this highly nutritious food. The current trend away from egg consumption may have contributed to chromium deficiencies. It is time to dispel the cholesterol/egg myth. The fact is that eating eggs is not responsible for high cholesterol levels. Again—just the opposite has been demonstrated. (Send for my "white paper" on eggs and cholesterol: Include a self-addressed stamped envelope and mail to: Nutrition, Box 2736, Novato, CA 94948. Write "eggs" on the outside of the envelope.)

Dr. Todd reports an interesting phenomenon that supports this view. A diabetic himself, Dr. Todd says that when he has two eggs for breakfast, he requires little or no insulin that day.[63]

Another example of the "low quantity/high absorption" phenomenon is represented by the minimal zinc content in breast milk compared with bottled milk. Babies who are breast-fed exhibit higher zinc levels than bottle-fed babies, in spite of the low measure of zinc in breast milk.[64] Eating intact, nature-designed food proffers benefits that cannot yet be explained.

The amount of chromium content indicated for each food listed above has been established under ideal conditions—hardly the status of the food in our kitchens. As you can see, foods with absorbable chromium have been highly processed or are the types of foods which are not generally consumed today. As if all this isn't disturbing enough, overheating of foods helps to form a chromium complex difficult to absorb.[65]

Since American cheese, beer, and wine are not likely to enhance your immune system, the number of wholesome foods comprising respectable amounts of chromium can be counted—as they say—on the fingers of one hand. And even those few foods are only slightly higher in chromium than most other foods. Dr. Todd of Waynesville, North Carolina, Dr. Rosenbaum of Corte Madera, California, Dr. Corsello of Huntington, New York, and many other nutrition-oriented physicians do not depend on high-chromium foods for their chromium-deficient patients, but rather on supplementation.

Given the foodways of our time, these physicians believe that eating a high-chromium diet for the sake of achieving desired chromium levels is not easy to come by. This does not mean that good dietary practices are to be ignored. The doctors just like to "tell it like it is; no false promises." SAD, the Standard American Diet, does not deliver enough chromium.

MENUS WHICH INCLUDE FROZEN, CANNED, AND OVERPROCESSED FOODS ARE NOT THE ANSWER TO CHROMIUM DEFICIENCIES.

CHROMIUM AS A SUPPLEMENT

It was after Dr. Mertz's discovery in 1959 that this amazing essential trace element became available in supplemental form. The forerunner consisted of simple, inorganic chromium salts such as chromium chloride, oxide, or acetate. The biological activity of these products was almost nonexistent. Some even proved to be toxic when used over a period of time.[66]

The next generation of chromium supplements surfaced in the early 1970s as amino-acid chelated chromium. (The word *chelate* means *to grab*; chelated nutrients "grab" or bind to other substances.) Amino-acid chelates appeared to revolutionize chromium supplementation by increasing absorption. But amino-acid chelated minerals are often high in vanadium, a chromium antagonist.[67] What's more, chelation technology is not an exact science. Only partial chelation takes place, resulting in significant amounts of free chromium salts. Often, so-called chelated minerals are merely crude mixtures of inorganic chromium and amino acids with very little biological activity. In addition, amino-acid chelated chromium is not in a form that insulin can readily use.

Next came yeast-based supplements. Although brewer's yeast is the richest source of GTF chromium, it typically contains less than two micrograms of chromium per gram of yeast, and less than half of this amount is in the biologically active GTF form.[68] So using brewer's yeast as a chromium source necessitates consuming large quantities to meet the daily requirement of 50 to 200 micrograms. A portion of food the size of a fist usually equals about 100 grams. A fist-sized portion of brewer's yeast would contain 200 micrograms of chromium. This is exactly what had been prescribed as a daily dose for diabetics in the last century.

A few decades ago, at the dawn of the nutrition movement in this country, the nutrition "gurus" suggested at least several tablespoons of brewer's yeast a day. (Among these wise prophets were Carlton Fredericks and Gaylord Hauser.) When my two sons were of grade school age, they had brewer's yeast races: each would grab a handful of tablets, and the winner was the one who swallowed the batch first. They went through school with almost perfect attendance records. We were convinced that brewer's yeast was a significant contributing factor to their good health.

Attempts to extract and concentrate GTF from brewer's yeast proved successful in the laboratory, but this method of extraction is impractical on a large scale. Although the chromium, as well as the GTF content, is substantially higher than that found in plain brewer's yeast, only about 25 percent of the chromium is actually complexed into the GTF form.

Chromium picolinate, a high-tech chromium compound, is another innovation, comprised of chromium bound to picolinic acid. This is a new product that does not have too much scientific validation in the medical literature as yet. Questions have been raised concerning the safety of picolinic acid since it has been identified as a niacin antagonist.[69]

Another yeast-free chromium complex, called *chromium polynicotinate*, consists of chromium bound to nicotinic acid (niacin). Recall that the chromium-niacin complex was identified by Dr. Mertz as the active component of the glucose tolerance factor.

THE CHEMICAL AND BIOLOGICAL ACTION
OF CHROMIUM POLYNICOTINATE
IS THE SAME AS
NATURALLY OCCURRING GTF.

Chromium polynicotinate was shown to lower blood glucose levels after only one hour or less—considerably more rapid than other forms tested.[70]

Everything I have ever learned from research and clinical experience confirms my belief that the *whole* is better than its parts when it comes to nutrition. The GTF chromium polynicotinate complex appears to resemble that which is natural more than other forms of available supplementation. When taken in this form, you spare your body the burden of conversion processes.

Pulitzer-prizewinning author René Dubos reminds us that *wherever human beings are concerned, trend is not destiny. We are reversible. We are not prisoners of our biological [or environmental] inheritance.*

THERE IT IS:
CHROMIUM, ALL-PURPOSE NUTRIENT!

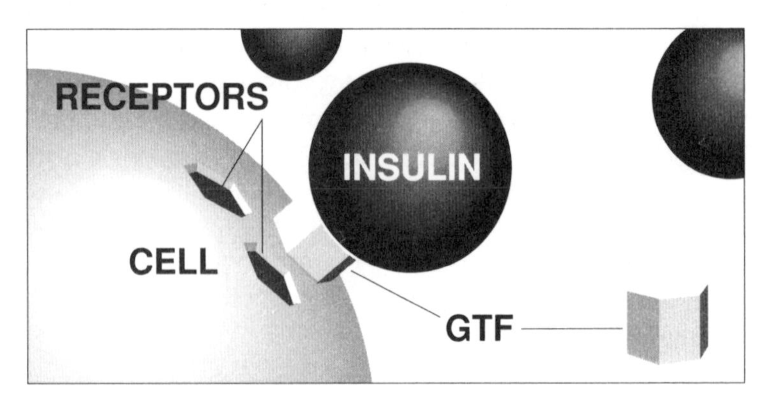

Figure 1. *GTF chromium binds insulin to cell membrane receptor sites. At these sites, insulin transports glucose and amino acids inside the cell. (Artist's conception.)*

CHAPTER 2

ENERGY

what it is, how you get it from food, from exercise and from supplements

---

GLOSSARY

ATP - adenosine triphosphate; chemical used by body to transfer energy derived from food to various forms of work, including muscular activity.

carbohydrates - starches and sugars present in most foods.

complex carbohydrates - foods containing large amounts of starches and sugars in their whole, unadulterated form—bonded with associated proteins, fiber, vitamins, minerals, and other nutrients; examples: vegetables, whole grains, nuts and seeds.

simple carbohydrates - carbohydrates broken down into more simple compounds, occurring in some foods naturally, but mostly caused by food processing (when food is taken apart); examples are honey, sucrose or fructose, and refined sugar.

endurance capacity - time taken to exercise to exhaustion, irrespective of mode of exercise.

energy - ability to work; power that can be translated into motion.

enzyme - protein, produced by a cell; acts as catalyst in biochemical reactions.

glycogen - complex carbohydrate formed from glucose in liver, serving as sugar reserve; can be converted back to sugar (glucose) and given up to blood; word means "sugar former."

mitochondria - very small structures found inside cells; center of enzyme activity.

oxidation - combination of substance with oxygen.

nutritional oxidation - break-down of food for energy use.

pyruvic acid - involved in generation of energy during muscle contraction.

to potentiate or *to spare insulin* - making insulin metabolism more efficient.

CHROMIUM AS AN ENERGY ENHANCER

If you want to win a gold medal, you have to select the right parents, or read books like this.

ENERGY: WHAT IT IS

Name the activity—*any* activity. My friend Esther is engaged in it. She directs plays and acts in them. She makes antique dolls, for which she sews exquisite and authentic costumes. Esther bakes unusual cakes for anyone's special event. She's an artist. And a teacher. And a world traveler. Despite her innumerable involvements and talents, she has time for those who need her, regardless of request. Esther's most unique attribute is her sparkle, spirit and spunk.

When I think of talent, I think of Esther. When I think of *energy*, I think of Esther. Esther knows so much about so many things. I wonder if she knows that her incredible gusto is in some way related to her chromium metabolism.

FROM FOOD TO FUEL

Would *you* like to have more energy? Most say, "Of course,"—not only those who require naps in the afternoon or the yuppie who falls away early evening, but also the energetic young jock who seems to have already harnessed all the vigor available. In fact, well-trained athletes near the top of the might-and-muscle continuum are the first to show interest in learning how to boost energy, one of life's greatest forces.

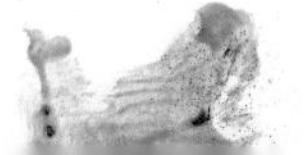

THE GOOD NEWS IS THAT ENERGY POWER CAN BE INCREASED AT ANY LEVEL WHETHER YOU ARE ATHLETIC OR LETHARGIC, OLD OR YOUNG, MALE OR FEMALE.

Your energy is inherent—your body makes it from the food you eat, and it does so with the use of a familiar process. It is the same chemistry that causes iron to rust and takes place when an apple turns brown after it is cut open. The action is called *oxidation*—the union of a substance with oxygen. Nutrients in your food are gradually broken down by this process, which is critical to your energy supply. Every sweep of your hand, every blink of your eye, is accomplished with the use of energy that once was the cereal you had for breakfast, your lunch sandwich, the fish filet you ate for dinner. The ultimate fate of the food you eat is to supply energy for your current and future needs.

DEFINING ENERGY

The definition of energy includes changes which help to transform one kind of energy to another. In this case, the energy in food is set free for your use when your food is oxidized. Part of the energy is for immediate needs, and the balance is saved for use later on. It's like having money in your wallet to meet present demands, with money in the bank for subsequent use. But part of the energy vanishes, in the sense that it cannot be recaptured and used again. (I guess we feel that way about some of our money, too!)

Surely you have read analogies which liken your body to a machine requiring fuel to keep it going. Comparisons of people-power are made with combustion engines in particular because of their similarities.

PEOPLE-POWER AND COMBUSTION ENGINES
• Energy for work is released by oxidation or burning of fuel. • Heat is a by-product of the release of that energy.

A machine, however, needs energy only when it is doing external work. You are never completely at rest. *Your body must work to live*. This is demonstrated by the fact that you are always warm, even when you sleep, and only in death is the body cold.

The energy required during an eight-hour period of sleep may be equal to the amount used by an inactive person during the day. The activity of your brain alone accounts for about one-fifth of the energy expended by your body at rest. Your liver and kidneys work constantly at cruising speed. Your nervous system continues to function as you sleep. And, of course, your energy expenditure accelerates during daily activities.

The business of ingesting food raises your energy output because a portion of energy is used to cover the energy "cost" of food metabolism. In other words, the very act of eating uses up energy. Cutting a pattern out of a piece of cloth is analogous. The material used for the garment can be likened to the production of energy, and the leftover scraps of material relate to the "cost" or heat lost.

Metabolism may be thought of as a process that begins where digestion ends. Food is *broken down* in digestion. But metabolism includes the changes that occur in the vital processes inside your cells—the transformation of the nutrients taken apart by digestion.

Some foods "cost" more than others—you pay for the energy needs of digestion and metabolism. Fat, for example, "costs" more than carbohydrates. (Perhaps the fabric has a striped motif, so that the fabric pieces can only be matched a certain way. Still more waste; the pattern requires more fabric because of its design, creating more "cost." So it is with fat.)

Your body cannot produce energy out of nothing. If you eat an insufficient amount of food to cover the cost of energy expended, some of your body tissues become the fuel, and you lose weight. Conversely, when you consume more food than you utilize for work and energy needs, you squirrel away added weight. Most of us can validate these facts with personal experience. (I can, many times over.)

BODY EFFICIENCY AND ENERGY

Did you ever wonder why you experience the feeling of heat while engaged in strenuous activity? To do a given amount of work, five times as much body fuel must be oxidized as would be represented by the work alone. In other words, only one-fifth of the fuel is altered into work energy, while about four-fifths appears as heat. It's as though five times the amount of fabric is left on the cutting room floor. (A Garment Center cutter would be fired for wasting so much cloth.)

This degree of "efficiency" with which your body makes energy is greater than that of a steam locomotive, less than that of a Diesel, but just about equal to that of a good automobile engine. In other words, a good auto engine also loses about four-fifths of its energy in heat, just as you do.

THE ENGINE OF YOUR CAR REQUIRES CONSTANT COOLING WHILE IT IS RUNNING, JUST AS YOU DO.

Although we only seem to be aware of this heat when we exercise energetically, heat production in smaller amounts is a steady by-product of any action involving work. (We can often explain our lost energy better than we can explain lost money.)

Sometimes, however, we function with even less efficiency, which means that work is accomplished at a greater cost—more fuel and oxygen are needed to produce a given amount of work, while a larger proportion of the energy appears as heat. So we may plod along with the more limited efficiency of the Little-Engine-That-Could (but almost couldn't) instead of the efficiency of the more competent automobile. It's no different than a company doing millions of dollars worth of business, but showing only a small percentage of profit,

Unlike an engine, you can adjust to your particular environment and varied needs. You can store surplus energy, and borrow from it as needed. Your energy is more or less "charged" ahead, ready to go, as in a wound-up spring or having money in the bank. Oxidation takes place after the work is over, in preparation for the next contraction—as though rewinding the spring, or recharging the battery. Your muscles can adapt to the effort and vary their efficiency under different circumstances. Under very special conditions, your energy competence can be increased from the average 20 percent to 33 percent—more like the Diesel, or a company showing a greater margin of profit.

INDIVIDUAL DIFFERENCES IN ENERGY

How many of you live with, or are close to, someone who eats an equivalent or greater amount of food than you consume, and yet remains as thin as the proverbial rail? (This has been my lot. Following dinner, my husband consumes the best snacks I ever watched! And he can still wear his World War II army uniform.)

Diverse energy efficiency is the reason why two people on identical diets respond uniquely to weight gain. Energy balance can be maintained on widely differing food intakes. British nutrition researcher, Dr. E. Widdowson, demonstrated this concept about three decades ago.

FOR ANY TWENTY PEOPLE OF THE SAME AGE, SEX, AND OCCUPATION, ONE INDIVIDUAL COULD BE FOUND WHO IS EATING TWICE AS MUCH AS ANOTHER AND SOME INFANTS EAT EVEN MORE THAN SOME ADULTS.[1]

Distinctions in energy efficiency are due to differences in heat production—variations which can arise from many causes, including stress, environmental temperature, commonly used drugs, hormonal imbalances, heredity, the type of work performed, previous training or practice, fatigue, and *your individual responses to food*.

The last factor is very significant. You lose some of your fuel through a possible inability to completely digest and absorb food, or to completely oxidize it in your tissues.

ENERGY IS DEPENDENT ON:

- the food you ingest
- the presence of important nutrients in that food
- the state of your digestive processes

You can see why we have a wide range of energy utilization. These facts also help to explain another phenomenon: people who stop eating foods to which they are sensitive report weight loss and energy gain.

It's interesting to note that this human variable is not usually found among animals, not even among animals that are domesticated.

STOREHOUSING ENERGY

Even if you are not chemistry-minded, the next few paragraphs may help to give you a cursory understanding of the force behind energy.

You know that food offers three main sources of energy:

(1) carbohydrates
(2) proteins
(3) fats

The word *carbohydrate* is suggested by the fact that carbohydrates are made up of the elements carbon, hydrogen, and oxygen. The word *hydrate* stems from the presence of hydrogen and oxygen in the same proportion as in water. (Remember H_2O from school science?) Carbohydrates are either sugars or more complex compounds such as starches—which are formed by the union of many sugars.

Here are the facts you should remember:

»The carbon, hydrogen, and oxygen atoms are linked in a molecule called *glucose*, which, as explained, is what much of your food turns into.

»Your blood must contain a specific amount of glucose at all times—no more, no less.

»The glucose level in your blood rises after eating, exceeding your body's needs.

»Your liver comes to the rescue: It functions as a storage and distribution center, having the ability to remove excess glucose from your blood—amounts not needed for energy at the moment.

»The oversupply is converted by your liver to form glycogen, allowing your blood level to settle back to normal.

»As blood-sugar levels drop below your requirement—which happens between meals—your body just doesn't sit around waiting for the next meal. As explained, you need that energy supply even if you are a couch potato, enjoying a siesta, goofing off, doing nothing. Your liver reconverts the stored glycogen to glucose, sending it back into your blood as needed.

»The conversion from glucose to glycogen keeps your body from being flooded with glucose after meals and from running short of glucose at other times.

Glycogen, although made from glucose, is a more complex structure. It takes on a form with many branches, more like a bush than a tree. This configuration prevents the glycogen from pouring out of your liver too easily; you are protected from losing your energy holdings unless and until necessary. In addition, the workings of many enzymes are required for the turnabout to take place, offering additional protection.

The entire transaction can be likened to a large supply of food you purchase. Because you shopped ahead, you have a surplus. So you freeze the extras. When necessary, the food is defrosted and takes its original form. Like the freezer, your liver acts as a reservoir. Both the food in your freezer and the glucose in your liver are held in abeyance in an altered form: the food is frozen; the glucose has been transformed to glycogen. But each is restored to its initial useful structure when required.

Unlike the freezing of foods, in which case *you* initiate the defrosting, the changeover of glycogen back to glucose is self-activated—just as the thermostat of a heating unit automatically calls for heat when the temperature of a room drops below a pre-set value. A great system—as long as nothing impairs its efficiency.

To a lesser extent, your muscles share the function of storing glycogen, but do so in smaller amounts. Muscle glycogen is especially useful to fuel the requirement of sudden and extreme spurts of energy for a few minutes at a time. This is important for intense, short-term activities such as sprints for the athlete, or the "fight-or-flight" reaction that most of us experience when confronted with a threatening situation. No time for defrosting now!

Liver glycogen is the only cache from which blood glucose is replenished. Muscle glycogen is not used for the back-to-glucose conversion—it cannot be reinstated in your blood.

Even though muscle contains about one percent glycogen compared with five-to-ten percent in your liver, all the muscle glycogen is available for rapid glucose conversion and immediate use should a red-alert energy response be necessary.[2]

THE RELEASE OF ENERGY

Unless you are in active athletic competition, you are inclined to take normal, every-day energy for granted. The actual production of energy is dazzling.

»Energy release begins with the division of the glucose molecule into two smaller molecules of pyruvic acid.

»These molecules then move to compartments of the cell known as *mitochondria*.

»Each mitochondrion musters up an astounding amount of activity. Considering its size, this is extraordinary: it is only a thousandth the size of the already microscopic cell.

»As heat is liberated, pyruvic acid molecules, small as they are, are taken apart in a progression of painstakingly rigorous steps which rely on a network of enzymes.

»Each enzyme fractures a particular bond, reducing the molecule—carbon atom by carbon atom.

»Energy is released with each of these splits—which now get stored in bonds of yet another chemical compound, *adenosine triphosphate* (ATP).

»Every glucose molecule yields many molecules of ATP. ATP can be broken down easily to release its energy as needed by the cell.

Think of all this going on as you do nothing more than turn the pages of this book, or get up from your chair to go to the fridge for a snack. Imagine the hustle and bustle created when you move more energetically, as in aerobics!

THE FOOD YOU EAT IS BARTERED FOR ACTION THROUGH THE MOLECULES OF ATP.

The process is complex, but all you really need to know is that *what you eat dictates the efficiency with which all this takes place*. Remember: energy efficiency can vary from 20 percent (or less) to as much as 33 percent. The more efficient, the more energy. Your lifestyle choices ultimately drive those little engines inside your cells.

THE RELEASE OF GLUCOSE DURING EXERCISE

As recently as two decades ago we learned that with intensified energy demands—whether you are jogging down the road, jazzercising in front of the TV, walking up and down steps, or running to catch a bus—the glucose output from your liver is increased. A group of Scandinavian researchers reported that animals performing endurance exercise (exercising to exhaustion) ceased to work as soon as the supply of glucose from their livers became depleted.[3] Similar responses have been observed in humans at the end of exercise periods, thereby limiting performance potential.

AS BLOOD GLUCOSE DECREASES, SO DOES PERFORMANCE.

The more glycogen stored in your muscles at the start of an activity, the more stamina you'll exhibit during your performance. There is, however, an upper limit beyond which no more glycogen is normally backlogged—just as your freezer has a finite capacity as a repository for food, or your gas tank for fuel.

And there isn't that much glucose to begin with. Compare the limited 450 grams (or approximately one pound) of glucose stored by your liver and muscles with your body's storage of fat. Fat takes up 12 percent of the male body, and 25 percent of the female body.[4] (That's about 20 pounds of fat if you're an average male, and about 30 if you are female.)

The fact that *decreased blood glucose restricts your energy level* is very significant. Low blood sugar means no energy reserve. This is the reason why your abilities are so confined when you are hungry, and why hypoglycemics are always so tired. In both cases, you "run out of steam." In both cases, your blood glucose is low. *Decreased blood glucose restricts your energy level.*

EFFECTS OF GLYCOGEN RESERVES

The pep and punch of many runners wanes after the first hour. Cross-country cyclists who have exhausted their glycogen reserves may find little difficulty in sustaining a reasonable pace on level ground, but they are no longer able to tackle even modest inclines. Glycogen capacity can be almost expended after 75 to 100 minutes of energetic endurance work. The amount of glucose used by a limb increases at least ten- to twenty-fold when exercising.[5] Since the amount of glycogen stored is trivial to begin with, *faster deterioration is most obvious in contestants who start out with low glycogen levels.*[6]

ENERGY SUMMARY
• You create energy from food you eat. • Your energy power can be increased at any level. • A specific amount of glucose is required in blood at all times. • Excess glucose is stored as glycogen. • The more glycogen stored, the more energy. • Glycogen is converted back to glucose as an energy source when needed. • Inefficient energy metabolism causes energy loss. • Efficient energy metabolism increases energy and increases endurance.

The ability to store, transport and use glucose results in a dramatic increase in energy and endurance—a goal which can be accomplished with a three-part program.

ENERGY: HOW YOU GET IT FROM FOOD

DOES A GLUCOSE FIX WORK?

If glucose is the basis of energy supply, it would appear that ingesting glucose, or foods containing glucose, could be a solution. Many studies show that this is not the case. One classic survey describes a group of runners given glucose in water 45 minutes prior to exercising on a treadmill. The runners "ran" on the treadmill for 30 minutes. Another group repeated the exercise, but was only given water. In the group that ingested glucose, muscle glycogen concentration was lower, endurance capacity was 19 percent less, and hypoglycemia developed.[7]

So, although glucose is the fuel that forms glycogen, glucose ingestion does not convert to glycogen to help you to attain more energy.

GLUCOSE INGESTION
DOES NOT IMPROVE ENDURANCE
NOR DOES IT DELAY EXHAUSTION.

Fructose, a sugar found in fruit and honey, has been recommended as a fuel because it maintains more stable blood glucose during exercise than glucose.[8] Fructose, however, produces no greater improvement in endurance.

THE SEARCH FOR ENERGY FOODS

If you can't bolster glycogen stores by eating sugar, the simple glucose, what is the secret for increasing these reserves? American athletes have long been told that all they have to do is abide by "the four food groups." Helen Guthrie, writing in the *Journal of Nutrition Education*, advises that the "basic four" does not even satisfy the nutrient needs of the average sedentary person, much less the vigorous athlete.[9]

Although it was only recently that researchers discovered the scientific links among diet, fitness, and endurance capacity, suspicion that some specific nutrient might confer superior vitality on the athlete is historical. People have been attempting to feed themselves "high test fuel" for optimal performance and the relief of fatigue for centuries. Records of this quest go back at least twenty-five hundred years. Dromeus, in 450 BC, theorized that muscle meat endowed the athlete with muscle strength. Five hundred years later, Plutarch recommended "light, thin" foods, like garden produce and fish with little fat. A university football team in the 1980s bankrupted its alumni fund because of its consumption of expensive royal jelly.[10]

Controlled studies surfaced in 1939, firmly establishing a relationship between a high-carbohydrate diet and improvement in endurance capacity. It was shown that when carbohydrate provided only 5 percent of the total energy intake, subjects could work at a standard load for a period of one hour. But with a 90 percent carbohydrate diet, the exercise time was quadrupled.[11]

During World War II researchers investigated whether or not diet could have a positive influence on performance and/or defer fatigue for aviators flying at high altitudes. It was shown that preflight meals rich in carbohydrate improved endurance. This was not true of meals rich in protein. Decreased efficiency in muscular work followed prolonged periods of low calorie intake. *Various personality changes* also became evident.[12]

Not much attention was paid to these results until 1967, when *Acta Physiologica Scandinavica* reported that energy capacity increases 300 to 400 percent when a diet is changed from carbohydrate-poor to carbohydrate-rich. A few athletes noticed, but not enough to make an impact.

IN 1979, IT WAS EXPLAINED THAT ENDURANCE FOR AEROBIC WORK CAN BE MAINTAINED AT DIFFERENT AVERAGES, DEPENDING ON THE DIET PRECEDING THE ACTIVITY.[13]

ENDURANCE AVERAGES FOR AEROBIC WORK
• one hour after a diet high in fat • three hours after a mixed diet • four hours after several days on a high carbohydrate diet

In 1981, the *American Journal of Clinical Nutrition* informed its readers that complex carbohydrates led to significantly higher muscle glycogen levels than a simple carbohydrate diet. *The heightened vitality was thought to be due to the increased glycogen stored in muscles associated with high carbohydrate diets.* Now everyone was at full attention. The vocabulary that turned the tide was: *more glycogen storage*. It was finally apparent that *carbohydrate most readily provides the kind of energy needed to activate muscles.*

COMPLEX CARBOHYDRATES BEFORE AN EVENT

Many studies concerning complex carbohydrates and performance increased our knowledge of glycogen metabolism. We learned the following:

»If you starve for twenty-four hours, your reserves of carbohydrates are exhausted.[14]

»If you eat carbohydrate-poor meals, you have the same low liver glycogen as you would have if you starved for twenty-four hours.[15]

»If you eat foods high in protein and fat for ten days, this also significantly reduces glycogen.

»A carbohydrate-rich diet results in an immediate increase in liver glycogen after only twenty-four hours.[15]

How can all this wisdom be applied? If several days are available for dietary preparation before an athletic event, *or* for a major house or office move, *glycogen reserves can be increased substantially by consuming complex carbohydrates.*

There is no longer any doubt that the amount of glycogen in your liver and muscles depends in large part on whether the supply of carbohydrate in your diet has been *liberal* or *scanty.*

Although overwhelming confirmation of the value of a complex carbohydrate diet continues to proliferate, people cling to their habits and find it difficult to "let go" of their usual food patterns.

RESULTS OF HIGH CARBOHYDRATE DIETS CONSUMED FOR A FEW DAYS PRECEDING AN EVENT
• long distance cyclists ride farther[16] • long distance cross country skiers race faster[17] • long distance canoeists paddle more rapidly[18] • soccer players score more goals in the latter part of matches because they maintain energy levels for a longer period of time[19]

THE SEARCH CONTINUES

As information about carbohydrates and endurance accumulates, so does that of an inverse relationship between fats and endurance capacity.[20] Unhealthful ratios of fats are easy to come by among fast-food-, steak-and-potato-, and gourmet-dining-consumers.

The researchers are still trying to put the puzzle pieces together in an effort to determine the best time and form of carbohydrate intake.

GLUCOSE AND THE THINKING ATHLETE

Glucose is not just for muscle power. An adequate *cerebral* supply of glucose is also important in sports requiring tactical thought. During sailing races, for example, competitors must be attentive to the trim of the boat and sails, changing wind and tides, tactical maneuvers, crew rapport, and must also anticipate future strategic moves by opponents. The crew of a small boat is particularly vulnerable to a fall in blood glucose, since sustained isometric contractions of the leg and abdominal muscles are needed when counterbalancing the vessel. (An isometric exercise is one in which a particular set of muscles is tensed for a period of seconds, in opposition to another set of muscles or an immovable object.)

A positive association between the resting blood glucose levels of dinghy sailors and the team captain's *rating of their performance* has been demonstrated by a serious Canadian sailor. Before allowing anyone to crew for him during competitions, this skipper now checks blood-sugar levels.[21]

Your brain depends on carbohydrate for its metabolism, so that as your blood sugar falls, the problem of central nervous system fatigue is added to the weakness of muscle fibers.[22]

We've established the importance of complex carbohydrates. Now let's clarify. Exactly what is a complex carbohydrate, and why does it help to supply more energy?

DEFINING COMPLEX CARBOHYDRATES: OXYGEN FOODS

Complex carbohydrates are vegetables, whole grains, seeds, and nuts. Note that fruits are not included in my list of complex carbohydrates. Yes, fruit meets the *classical* definition of a complex carbohydrate, but the content of simple sugars in fruits is high—very high. Fruit is not equal in value to energy-inducing vegetables and whole grains. (See Chapter 8 for an optimum ratio of fruit-to-vegetable consumption.)

Complex carbohydrates can be further divided into starchy and fibrous varieties. The starchy carbohydrates help to build size and strength, and include white potatoes, sweet potatoes, brown rice, peas, oatmeal, corn and tomatoes. The fibrous category serves to create lean bodies, and includes asparagus, broccoli, cabbage, carrots, cauliflower, celery, lettuce, and spinach.

Dr. Stephen Levine points out that complex carbohydrates have 16 parts of oxygen and only 14 parts of carbon and hydrogen. He explains:

More than half of a complex carbohydrate is oxygen, but the percentage of oxygen in fats is less than 10 or 15 percent, so fats are very low in oxygen. In fact, fats are oxygen "robbers" because they require so much oxygen to be metabolized. Protein is composed of 20 to 50 percent oxygen, depending on the specific amino acid profile. It is obvious: complex carbohydrates have the most oxygen.[23]

One reason that complex carbohydrates help to maintain higher levels of performance may be related to their high oxygen content. Far less heat is liberated when carbohydrates are burned for fuel, so there is greater efficiency in the energy-creating process. Fat foods may cost more to metabolize because they are low in oxygen. This depletes oxygen supplies, and, consequently, less energy is available. Because extra oxygen is needed for their burning, a great deal of heat is released, changing your efficiency quotient.

THE FIRST CLUE FOR MORE ENERGY
IS THE CONSUMPTION OF
COMPLEX CARBOHYRATES.

Complex carbohydrates:

- improve endurance capacity during continued exercise
- help to regain muscle glycogen more rapidly after a period of prolonged activity[24]
- are a good source of vitamins and minerals (in contrast to simple sugars)
- contain fiber (improving transit time)

Although offering protection against nutritional deficiencies, *complex carbohydrates do not insure total security for the athlete.* Read on.

ENERGY: HOW YOU GET IT FROM EXERCISE

THE SECOND CLUE FOR MORE ENERGY

Basic nutrition needs do not vary with activity. Nor, for that matter, are they different for inactive people. Experts generally agree that the same dietary principles that promote good health for the public at large maximize performance for most athletes. Metabolic processes, however, work more efficiently for the exerciser than the sedentary because a larger percentage of food is properly digested and assimilated. Given the same amount of food, the exerciser derives greater benefit than the couch potato. Better nutrient absorption increases energy level.

But there is a warning. Vitamin and mineral deficiencies

are not uncommon among athletes.[25] The athlete, for example, is at special risk for chromium deficiency, yet chromium is essential for the expanded energy needs.[26] *The effect of chromium deficiency is particularly deleterious for athletes because of their jacked-up energy requirements.* It's a Catch-22 situation: chromium is essential for exercise, and exercise causes chromium depletion.

Aerobic activity mobilizes chromium into circulation, which encourages utilization and excretion. A study carried out by the United States Department of Agriculture shows that chromium losses increase nearly five times the normal amount following a six-mile run, and excretion doubles on an exercise day compared with a non-exercise day.[27] Sugar and refined carbohydrate, mainstay foods for many athletes, also cause chromium waste.

EXERCISING IS THE SECOND CLUE FOR MORE ENERGY.

The reason glucose is taken from your bloodstream during exercise is to provide fuel for energy. After exercise, or when sedentary, glucose is used to rebuild your muscle glycogen stores.[28] Recall that human energy is prepared ahead, ready to go. *Chromium helps insulin move the needed glucose into your cells.* This is the process that transports glucose to where it is actually utilized for tissue generation. Unfortunately, once chromium is applied in this way, about 95 percent is then excreted. The small balance returns to storage.[29]

The good news is that understanding this biochemical phenomenon highlights the way to solving the energy dilemma.[30]

HOW TO GET ENERGY FROM SUPPLEMENTS

THE THIRD CLUE FOR INCREASED ENERGY

In addition to complex carbohydrates and exercise, you may benefit from supplements. The point to remember is that exhaustion can be caused by a shortage of fuel.[31]

»One study with test animals, reported in *Poultry Science*, involved two sets of animals. Each was fed the same diet, but only one group received chromium supplementation. The results demonstrated that supplementing with chromium significantly increased liver glycogen concentrations.[32]

»Other research shows similar results: chromium supplementation produces much greater glycogen formation and thereby greater concentration in tissues from the available glucose.[33]

»Chromium supplementation not only enhances muscle and heart glycogen, but also bone and kidney chromium concentrations.[34]

There is no longer doubt about the incredible relationship between chromium nutrition and performance competence.

THE THIRD CLUE FOR MORE ENERGY
IS CHROMIUM POLYNICOTINATE.

If you want to win a gold medal, you have to select the right parents, or read books like this. But what if you aren't an athlete, or even committed to simple aerobics? Active or not, chromium metabolism is beneficial because of its effect on your glycogen stores, thereby delaying fatigue.

SUMMARY

Without chromium, energy production comes to a screeching halt. Following a high carbohydrate meal, insulin and GTF chromium are released into your blood stream to facilitate glucose metabolism. GTF chromium is responsible for attaching insulin to cell membrane receptor sites. Insulin is responsible for transporting glucose inside the cell where it is metabolized into energy. Thanks to GTF-mediated insulin, glucose transport inside your cell is increased fifteen- to twenty-fold.

GTF chromium and insulin serve as workers shuttling glucose in and out of cells. When blood glucose is elevated and energy demands are minimal, GTF-insulin stores glucose in the form of glycogen. When energy demands are increased, GTF-insulin breaks down glycogen into glucose, which is burned for energy. But without GTF chromium, glucose metabolism is severely impaired.

Researchers at the United States Department of Agriculture proved that insulin alone has little effect on glucose metabolism. But in combination with GTF-chromium, glucose is rapidly transported inside the cell where it is metabolized into energy.

For a *new you*, it's a triumvirate:

(1) Consume intact food in the form of complex carbohydrates.
(2) Get into an aerobic exercise program (just enough, don't overdo).
(3) Take a small amount of chromium supplementation.

THERE IT IS:
GTF CHROMIUM FOR THE SLUGGISH
OR THE ATHLETE

Insulin alone is ineffective . . .

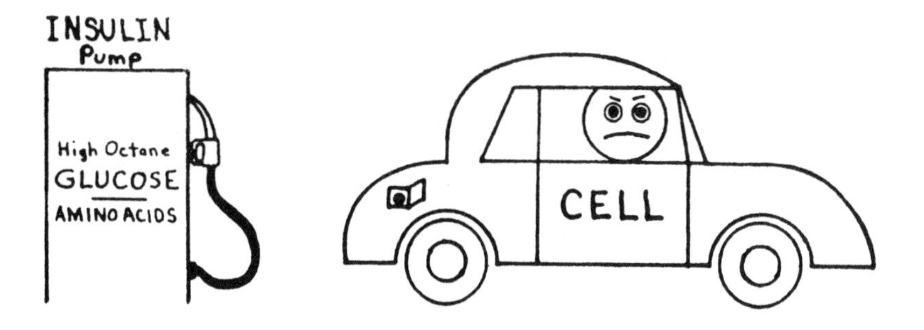

. . . but with GTF, insulin rapidly transports glucose and vital amino acids inside cells for energy and tissue generation.

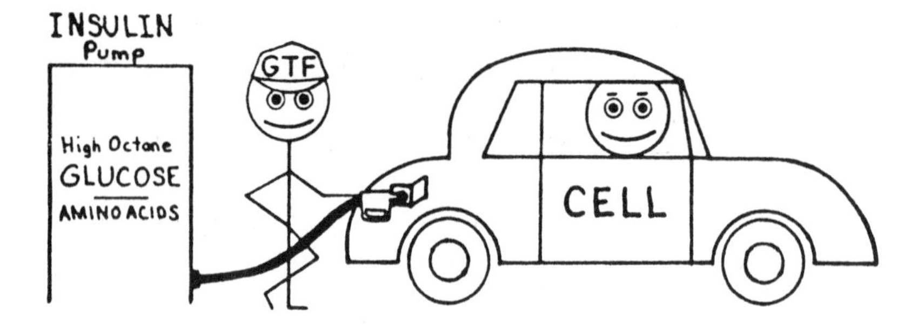

CHAPTER 3

FITNESS

what it is, what affects it, how body builders maintain it

GLOSSARY

anabolic - building complex compounds from simple ones in living organisms; opposite of catabolic.

catabolic - degradation of nutrient molecules into smaller and simpler end products.

growth hormone - hormone which stimulates growth, directly influencing protein, fat, and carbohydrate metabolism.

muscle fiber - structural cell of muscle.

steroids - any of a large group of compounds having specific physiological action.

CHROMIUM AS A FITNESS PROMOTER

As the athlete gropes for that competitive edge, he or she is very vulnerable to accepting bizarre and often dangerous fitness-building practices.

FITNESS: WHAT IT IS

The adjective *fit* has several meanings: *adapted, prepared, proper, worthy, ready, healthy.* The derivative noun, *fitness,* has become a buzzword, meaning the state of being in good physical shape. The fact that nutrients in general relate to fitness is not new. That chromium in particular has such a profound influence on fitness has only recently been explored scientifically. *Fitness* really means having a "never-felt-better" frame of mind; blooming, hearty and hale, bursting with vigor; waking up fresh as a daisy, and retiring with a relaxed sense of fatigue. I hope this describes *you.* If it doesn't, it can!

AN IMPORTANT TIP FOR EVERYONE

Here's a fitness tip for everyone in general and growing children, pregnant women, athletes and body builders in particular: when you consume sugar-laden foods for dinner, or eat sweet desserts after that meal and during the evening, you undermine your energy on two counts:

(1) The ingestion of high-sugar foods makes your chromium level drop. You already know the consequences: *Stressing your chromium requirements affects insulin efficiency and glucose metabolism.*

(2) Growth hormone is released during sleep. A high sugar food consumed late in the day blocks the nocturnal release of this hormone, thereby interfering with very important anabolic and energy responses.[1]

One of the concepts explored here is how these facts impact on your fitness level.

WISDOM FROM ANTIQUITY

It was just an old saying—very old—and only the macho paid attention. But now, "little old ladies in tennis shoes" (like many of my friends) and healthy young men and women who have sedentary jobs (like many of their children) are highly conscious of this Hippocratic truth, stated more than 2000 years ago:

All parts of the body which have a function, if used in moderation and exercised in labors in which each is accustomed, become thereby healthy, well developed, and age more slowly, but if unused and left idle they become liable to disease, defective in growth, and age quickly.[2]

Hippocrates was referring to moving your muscles (perhaps all 650 of them) to attain and maintain fitness. He knew that fitness could be achieved through good food and exercise. You know that, too, but you should know it as a way of life, not just as a platitude.

THE CHANGING EXERCISE SCENE

After World War II, it was a challenge to find enough runners for a single national marathon event. Now the Reeboks and Nikes pound pavements every day of the year from the rural lane in the country to city streets everywhere. Trained athletes competing in the San Francisco Bay-to-Breakers race crash through the finish line, seven and a half miles later, long before most of the huge crowd of 150,000 additional participants work their way to the start. Promoting fitness through exercise and sports has swung much more sharply into focus.

Ludwig Prokop, representing the Medical Commission of the International Olympic Committee in Vienna, Austria, stated:

Everything that is optimal for high-performance athletes as regards their performance and health must also prove necessary and beneficial for the fitness of regular people.[3]

Interest in fitness metabolism is expanding in direct proportion to the involvement in "working out." In spite of widespread advice and curiosity, however, studies show that few athletes follow the best dietary pattern for optimal sports performance. They generally eat too much fat and protein at the expense of carbohydrate.[4]

Minor nutritional inadequacies, not necessarily caused by lack of food, interfere seriously with high fitness and the level of functional capacity. As the athlete gropes for that competitive edge, he or she is very vulnerable to accepting bizarre and often dangerous fitness-building practices.

FITNESS: WHAT AFFECTS IT

CHROMIUM AND EXERCISE: SAME BENEFITS

We all know that exercise has specific beneficial effects. Here's exciting news: *the scientists at the United States Department of Agriculture have determined that the salutary reactions influenced by exercise are similar to those invoked by chromium.* For example:

»Exercise increases muscle sensitivity to insulin. So does chromium.[5]

»Exercise increases the ability to regulate blood glucose. So does chromium.[6]

»Exercise improves blood lipid profiles. So does chromium.[7]

So exercise and chromium are the cake *and* the icing. The researchers add that the availability of chromium in usable amounts and forms can be a rewarding and controlling factor during and after exercise.[8] This combination may in fact help add life to years, not just years to life. It translates to *fitness.*

RESTORING GLYCOGEN

While you are exercising, your muscle cells are busily combusting nutrients to create the energy required. This demolition is called *catabolism*, the tearing down of molecules into smaller and simpler end products—including the transition of glycogen back to glucose. (Recall that glycogen is the more complex structure; glucose the simpler one.)

After exercise your metabolism takes a 180-degree turn. The recovery period involves a switch from the catabolic response to *anabolic* reactions—that is, the building-up process. Among other reconstruction assignments, you resurrect the cargo in your muscles—in preparation for future need. Blood-born glucose is delivered to restock muscle and liver glycogen, which ultimately increases muscle mass.

Surprisingly, the anabolic phase of muscle-building is not exactly a reversal process. Suppose you take a very large and heavy stone and push it down from the top of a steep hill. The stone rolls downhill in a fairly direct pathway. But you may not be able to lug the stone back up to the top of the hill using precisely the same pathway taken in its descent. Some parts of the uphill climb may be similar, but you would probably have to follow another pathway with an incline that would not be as steep. In the same way, catabolic reactions are "downhill," and anabolic are "uphill." It's a lot easier for catabolic reactions to take place in your muscles than it is for the anabolic processes.[9] (Sorry about that.) All the more reason you want to supply the armamentarium to expedite and facilitate the mission.

IT IS EASIER FOR YOUR BODY
TO BREAK DOWN MUSCLE
THAN IT IS TO BUILD IT UP.

THE TRAINED VS UNTRAINED ATHLETE

Needless to say, the average trained athlete is generally in better shape than the nonathlete. Note these differences between trained and untrained individuals:

»Well-exercised muscles pick up glucose for the purpose of glycogen repletion more quickly than nonexercised muscles. The reason for this is that nonexercised muscles have a more difficult time responding to insulin.[10]

»Chromium excretion of trained athletes is significantly lower than that of untrained athletes, and is actually related to the degree of fitness.[11]

»Trained athletes oxidize more fat and less carbohydrate than the untrained when exercising at the same intensity.[12] The greater the aerobic fitness of an individual, the greater the contribution of fat metabolism to energy expenditure. This results in a more economical use of the limited glycogen stores, thereby delaying the onset of fatigue.[13]

»Thiamin and vitamin C stores are significantly lower in amateur athletes than in elite athletes.[14] (*Elite* refers to well-trained, competing athletes.) This is probably true of other nutrients as well.

But here are a couple of unexpected similarities among the trained and untrained:

»Forty percent of all food consumed by *both* trained and untrained athletes is fat.[15] Fat takes longer to leave your stomach. It is not a source of instant energy, and should be avoided in any pre-game meal. You do need a little fat, but a little goes a long way. And of course you need the right kind of fat, but that's another book.

»Any mild dehydration leads to decreased endurance and tumble-down performance for both the trained and untrained.

If we could get the trained athletes to improve their diets, and the nonathletic to move their butts, we would have a phenomenal improvement in this nation's fitness status.

Meanwhile, without making any other change, it appears that each group may benefit from supplementation with GTF chromium.

FITNESS: HOW BODY BUILDERS MAINTAIN IT

THE USE OF SYNTHETIC STEROIDS

Muscle fiber is unique in that its metabolic rate can be varied to a greater extent than the metabolic rate of the cells of any other tissue.[16]

WITH THE RIGHT PLANNING, YOU CAN DEVELOP MUSCLES TO YOUR LIKING.

Just think of the muscles you would have if you could exercise endlessly without either the catabolic effects or fatigue. But as you know, exhaustion is caused by a limitation of available fuel.[17]

Body builders work hard to look good. Expensive gyms, special equipment, first class training techniques, select supplements, unusual diets, and dangerous steroids have all been tried, and tried again. Taking steroids produces effects that are similar to those of repetitive muscular work. But there's no free lunch. Synthetic anabolic hormones can be hazardous. Your body answers very differently to isolated substances than it does to the same elements prepared or consumed in the context of intact food.

Global publicity has called attention to the disadvantages of steroids. Reactions include acne, liver damage, cataracts, heart disease, and uncontrollable "steroid rage," a condition of explosive, aggressive behavior caused by the effect of the steroids on certain areas of the brain. Adolescent boys show stunted bone growth.

These are the particular responses for men on steroids:

»smaller testicles
»lower sperm count
»infertility

These are the particular responses for women on steroids:

»balding
»facial hair growth
»permanently deepened voice[18]

When synthetic steroids are discontinued, muscles fall back to the status of pre-steroid use. *There are better ways to build muscle.* You don't have to do it at the expense of your health.

INSULIN: ANABOLIC HORMONE?

Because of its strong association with diabetes and the pancreas, it may surprise you to learn that insulin is referred to as an *anabolic* hormone. But without insulin, muscles won't grow.[19] In fact, insulin has the same effect on protein metabolism as it does on carbohydrate metabolism. Protein formation is actually disabled when insulin is not available or is ineffective; the catabolism of proteins increases, and protein production meets an impasse.

It turns out that insulin is not only essential for growth, but is your body's chief promoter of energy. For this reason, the importance of insulin has attracted the attention of experts in the field of physical development. Insulin has a direct effect on muscle cell membranes—facilitating glucose transport. Glucose cannot penetrate the cell walls unless it is attached to the insulin molecule.

Have you ever been on a merry-go-round and tried reaching for the ring, but to no avail? You keep going round and round, like the glucose in your blood, trying unsuccessfully to grasp that ring. Finally, you get off—just as the glucose that doesn't enter your cells is eventually excreted. (Not all the excess glucose is excreted. Some of it may be converted to precursors of fats called triglycerides, which can eventually become incorporated into fatty tissue.) If only your arms were longer, or you had some kind of appliance or tool crafted for the job.

Insulin significantly increases the transport of glucose from your blood into your muscles. This can dramatically affect a bodybuilder's energy supply. But how does insulin reach the ring? Chromium is just the tool! Chromium builds a "bridge" between the insulin molecule and the cell membrane.[20]

IN THE PRESENCE OF SUFFICIENT AMOUNTS OF CHROMIUM IN A SUITABLE FORM, LOWER QUANTITIES OF INSULIN ARE REQUIRED.[21]

Because of this progression of actions, chromium has been called a natural steroid alternative. GTF chromium may be the most efficient, most healthful, and least expensive way to build muscle. Remember, *insulin is your body's own anabolic hormone, and chromium potentiates insulin.*[22]

Noting the devastating effects of steroids, you can see why athletes are now taking GTF chromium supplements as a safe substitute.

In summary, insulin, with the help of chromium, acts as a shuttle that picks up the blood glucose and facilitates its entry through your cell membrane and right into your cell's interior.

COMPLEX CARBOHYDRATES AND MUSCLE

But what happens when you eat apple pie or strawberry short cake? The simple sugars in these foods set off hormones that roam through target tissues, causing insulin levels to increase. This helps to *restrain* the rise of glucose. *Insulin response is very dependent on the kind of carbohydrate consumed.*[23] (More about the deleterious effects of high insulin levels in Chapter 7.)

Complex carbohydrates (vegetables, whole grains, nuts and seeds) are the main source of muscle bulk and size because they load your muscle with glycogen.[24] (Cows build large quantities of muscle, yet they graze on grass.) Recall that eating a carbohydrate-rich diet after glycogen-depleting exercise significantly increases your muscle-glycogen stores. Liver glycogen is also optimized, increasing endurance. Such a diet provides a protein-sparing effect.[25]

EXERCISE AND INSULIN RESISTANCE

Taking two grams of carbohydrate per kilogram of body weight immediately after exercise results in a 300 percent increase in the rate of glycogen synthesis in the first two hours of recovery after exercise. (This would be about two portions of food for someone of average weight.)

»Delaying the ingestion of carbohydrate by two hours slows the rate of glycogen production by 47 percent.

»The reduced rate is caused by increased muscle insulin resistance developing during the first two hours of recovery![26]

Insulin resistance refers to the fact that insulin is present to escort glucose to your cells, but your cells refuse to admit the glucose. The bridge has not been built. (Insulin resistance is explained in Chapter 4.) *So part of the muscle-building plan is to have portions of complex carbohydrates at the ready for consumption immediately following your exercise endeavor.*

Athletes often reserve their peak pace for the latter part of a long event knowing that the rate of glycogen use is greatest during early stages. Energy stores are limited, but glycogen provides a convenient energy *reserve* for muscle because large quantities of fuel can be stockpiled in this form.

WARNINGS ABOUT INSULIN SHOCK

Over-zealous athletes have attempted to experiment by injecting insulin directly into the blood stream. This practice is life-threatening. Oral GTF chromium supplementation in recommended doses is safe; insulin injection for those with normal blood glucose is not.

Insulin applied intravenously causes an immediate drop in blood sugar. Too much can scavenge nearly all traces of glucose, causing your brain and central nervous system to shut down, resulting in insulin shock. Insulin shock can lead to unconsciousness, coma, and even death. Steroids may kill you slowly. Insulin injections can end your life *just like that*. There is no second chance.

Taking additional insulin is of no benefit anyway. It does not create a super-carbohydrate load, or build more muscle. Excess insulin creates imbalances in other hormone systems, making your entire metabolism go askew. In fact, high blood insulin causes you to cash in your chromium stores.

CHROMIUM AND GLYCOGEN REPLENISHMENT

It cannot be over-emphasized that chromium is a major key to insulin's benefits. Insulin is useless without it.[27]

RECOVERY FROM ANY PHYSICAL WORK IS HIGHLY DEPENDENT ON GLYCOGEN REPLENISHMENT.

The rate of resynthesis of glycogen is relatively slow; one or two days is needed for the full replenishment of glycogen stores.[28] Note that major league pitchers require a few days rest between their high-energy responsibilities.

So if you want to be "muscle-man," no cheating allowed, particularly after dinner. Energy depends on glycogen, which depends on insulin, which depends on GTF chromium. *For the want of a horse shoe nail....*

GROWTH HORMONE AND INSULIN

Growth hormone, a substance produced by your pituitary gland, has important functions that relate to glucose, insulin, and muscle.

GROWTH HORMONE
• stimulates the growth of muscle • strengthens ligaments and tendons • increases bone thickness

Glucose triggers the release of growth hormone.[29] Most athletes are familiar with this anabolic action, and also with that of testosterone. Less widely known is the fact that *growth hormone requires insulin to promote bigger muscles effectively.*[30]

> EXPERIMENTS SHOW THAT INSULIN ITSELF IS JUST AS ESSENTIAL FOR GROWTH AS GROWTH HORMONE AND TESTOSTERONE. LACK OF INSULIN ACTUALLY CAUSES A BREAKDOWN OF MUSCLE TISSUE.

Unlike growth hormone and testosterone, insulin influences the metabolism of *all* the body fuels.[31] When young animals are deprived of the glands which secrete growth hormone and insulin, their normal growth stops. If these animals are then injected with either growth hormone or insulin alone, a slight increase in growth occurs. But when both growth hormone and insulin are administered simultaneously, growth is dramatic. Each of these hormones promotes the cellular uptake of different amino acids.

INSULIN AND AMINO ACIDS

During the first few hours following a meal—when excess amino acids are available from the food you eat—proteins are manufactured, stored, and converted to your body tissues. Insulin is essential for this process.

FUNCTIONS OF INSULIN
IN AMINO ACID METABOLISM

- Insulin increases the uptake of vital amino acids by your cells.
- Insulin increases the synthesis of RNA and DNA, the genetic "blueprints" used to organize amino acids into proteins, which in turn form your body's tissues.
- Insulin inhibits the breakdown of proteins, thereby decreasing the tendency of muscle cells to break down their protein structure during exercise.[34]

When insulin is not available or is not working properly (for example, if there is a chromium deficiency), protein formation comes to a complete halt. When protein synthesis stops, the breakdown of protein increases (catabolism), and large quantities of amino acids are dumped into your blood where they are burned up for energy or converted to glucose.[35] That means less protein for lean muscle mass.

TEST YOURSELF:
TRY CHROMIUM SUPPLEMENTATION

If you feel like something the cat dragged in more often than not, your metabolic delivery may not be working efficiently. The right precursors can help you make and utilize your own natural insulin. *You can catch those rings.* You may want to test this very simply: with both your physician's approval and the guidelines set by the National Academy of

Science's recommended dietary allowances, follow the safe chromium supplementation strategy outlined in Chapter 8. See for yourself whether or not your energy capacity increases with the use of GTF chromium. Chances are you will be pleasantly surprised.

WHAT ABOUT AMINO ACIDS AND MUSCLE?

The effect of exercise on protein has been studied for many years, yet questions still remain. We all know that weight-lifting and other muscle sports increase muscle mass. Distance running, although it causes little or no size change, is responsible for other alterations in muscle tissue. These adaptations are the result of adjustments in protein metabolism.

Today's experts cite several reasons for encouraging athletes to emphasize supplementation with GTF chromium rather than increasing protein intake:

»Amino acids are often consumed in plentiful amounts by most people. Body builders in particular are usually well supplied with protein.

»Vigorous sports do not cause a persistent increase in the breakdown of protein.

»Protein in the form of supplements add nothing to performance.[36]

»Protein does not provide a significant fuel for energy or performance during exercise in healthy individuals.[37]

»Overdosing on protein increases the load on liver and kidney systems. It also encourages calcium loss.[38]

»Because it has highly specific dynamic actions, protein increases oxygen consumption.[39]

»Chromium is absolutely essential for muscle growth and energy production. Most athletes appear to be at risk for chromium deficiency.

Of course protein is important, but even those involved in the meat business agree with these precepts. A recent publication of the National Live Stock and Meat Board Research Department stated that the elite athlete requires little more protein than is recommended in the RDAs.[40] Chromium, on the other hand, is usually inadequate and is utilized and excreted as a result of exercise.

It is generally accepted that protein needs for active individuals are greater than those for inactive people. But there is little evidence to suggest that the massive quantities of protein routinely consumed by some athletes (even the weight-lifters!) are either necessary or beneficial.[41] What may be more pertinent is the fact that some amino acids are utilized to a greater extent than others during exercise. So, despite a high-protein diet, an exerciser may be protein-deficient. That's the reason good performance depends on a small amount of quality protein (foods that have complete amino acids in the right ratios), along with a large carbohydrate menu at every meal, described in detail in Chapter 8.

MUSCLE AND SEX DIFFERENCES

Muscle in women appear to be better equipped for aerobic metabolism than muscle in men. That's because the surface area of the total amount of aerobic-type muscle fibers is larger in women. Male muscle seems to be suited for activities where brief, powerful contractions are needed, such as that of power lifting.

Women have more fat—25 percent of total body mass, compared with 12 percent for males. Roger Bannister (of four-minute-mile fame) suggests that this difference is evolutionary: women require energy output over prolonged periods of labor during childbierth, but man as hunter was concerned with an explosive burst of speed over a very short time.[42] Natural sex steroid hormones may also contribute to these differences.

The trainability of muscle strength reaches a peak in early adult life. Muscular endurance can be increased more in children aged twelve to fifteen than in men, but men are more trainable than women.[43]

DIETING AND LEAN MUSCLE MASS

Insulin also participates in a number of control mechanisms that affect your weight and what happens to lean muscle mass when you lose weight. This, too, is of particular importance to the training athlete. Dieters may throw off lean muscle mass as fast or faster than fat.

> MORE THAN HALF THE WEIGHT LOST WHILE DIETING MAY BE LEAN MUSCLE TISSUE, IMPAIRING YOUR ABILITY TO KEEP WEIGHT OFF.

While Jack Sprat's low calorie diet causes *insulin depletion*, muscle tissue of his overweight wife is usually *insulin-resistant*.[32] For different reasons, they are both in trouble, winding up with similar energy-depleting problems.

By inhibiting the breakdown of lean muscle mass, insulin helps to maintain the integrity of your body's chief calorie-burning tissue. Insulin also appears to enhance functional thyroid status, the primary regulator of your body's basal metabolism, and the generator of a potent fat-burning hormone called *triiodothyronine*.[33]

WARNINGS CONCERNING CARBOHYDRATE-LOADING

Carbohydrate-loading programs were designed for the purpose of storing glycogen. A widely accepted exercise and dietary procedure for producing energy is called *glycogen supercompensation*. It involves exercising to exhaustion to lower muscle glycogen concentration, followed by three days on a low-carbohydrate diet (mainly fat and protein), followed by three days on a high-carbohydrate diet. This kind of yo-yo carbohydrate unloading and loading is *not* in your best health interest.

Despite the positive relationship between initial glycogen concentration and endurance performance, there are apprehensions about glucose supercompensation. Three days on a low-carbohydrate diet are not only unpleasant, but may also undermine your confidence if you are preparing for a competition. Furthermore, if you continue to exercise during the "low-carbo" days, there is danger of exercise-induced hypoglycemia—there just isn't enough carbohydrate to supply the needed glucose.[44]

Controlled studies showing increased stamina as a result of carbohydrate loading have only been done with men. And beneficial results are usually obtained for cycling only, not for running.[45]

THE NIACIN CONNECTION

The World Health Organization made some observations about high levels of physical activity: when involved in such activity for hours, niacin is among the few additional nutrients that should be elevated.[46] So, a safe way to increase insulin's powerful anabolic effects is through proper diet (those wonderful oxygen-rich complex carbohdrates), exercise, and GTF chromium/niacin complexed supplementation, *chromium polynicotinate.* (Chapter 8 details a supplement strategy for optimal performance.)

SUMMARY

You can see that energy expended during exercise is tightly regulated by very complex, but highly integrated, responses. A note to muscle-builders: remember that strenuous exercise leads to increased chromium needs and losses, but that excretion is lower in *trained* individuals. With increasing intensity of exercise, the reliance on fat utilization decreases and carbohydrate becomes the dominating energy source.[47] *Would you believe this information has been known for a hundred years?*

The glucose/glycogen/muscle connection is a lesson in interdependence. These are fascinating unconsciously coordinated acts, with the operation of each part governed by the state and function of the other parts.

Ultimately, what you put in your mouth and how you move your body pulls the reigns for these intricate mechanisms. The consequences bounce back in the form of energy, and either you are, (1) off and running or, (2) feeling like a wet rag. Chances are you are somewhere in-between. That, for most of us, is not enough. But now you know: There is a way to "pull up."

Athletes, however, must be realistic. The search for the specific magic substance that creates superior athletic performance and builds Atlas muscles reminds me of the ancient alchemists looking for the secret formula that changes lead to gold. Although chromium has a significant impact on your muscles, don't expect chromium alone to produce quick, dramatic, artificial muscle gains—the kind experienced with massive doses of synthetic steroids. Dr. Robert Brucker, chief toxicologist of Centinela Medical Center in southern California, warns about exaggerated claims made for certain chromium products.

Dr. Richard Anderson, of the United States Department of Agriculture, is a great proponent of chromium supplementation. He, too, has looked askance at reports indicating very quick, steroid-type muscle growth with its use. "I had a hard time believing such reports," stated Dr. Anderson, "especially after consulting with exercise physiologists." Because of the paucity of information, Dr. Anderson expects the United States Department of Agriculture to repeat studies making such claims.

Patience is necessary, and in the long term, the outcome should be even more exciting. *Adding GTF chromium polynicotinate may improve your overall health status.* If you stop taking chromium, your muscle growth won't disappear as it does when you discontinue steroids.

Although most of this discussion has been based on impaired physical energy, glucose deficiency also contributes to less proficiency at sedentary jobs—just as it interferes with the thinking sailor's abilities.[48] (See page 52.)

It should also be noted that the amount of glucose required for use in specific brain regions of older people does not differ from that of younger individuals.[49] The inventory of chromium, however, has diminished with age.

The subjects of energy and fitness are intricate. I've made no mention of norepinephrine, which decreases insulin, the counterregulatory hormones such as glucagon and epinephrine, or free fatty acids as fuel regulators. I've only touched on adenosine triphosphate (ATP) and pyruvic acid.

Those interested in more in-depth study can refer to the literature in the reference sections. The salient point demonstrated here is that chromium impacts on energy and fitness, and that the biological effect of GTF chromium on glucose metabolism is much greater than that of any inorganic chromium compound; thus the current and quickly-expanding use of GTF chromium by athletes. Supplementation should be seriously considered, not only by those who regard themselves as athletes, but also by anyone exercising on a regular basis—*and that should be almost everyone*. (Consult your physician.)

As Ludwig Prokop, of the International Olympic Committee Medical Commission, Vienna, Austria, says:

Sports put such high demands on people that all ways and means of supplementing physical training must be fully and consistently utilized to preserve health and improve psychosomatic fitness.[50]

Suffice it to say that supplementing with chromium may stoke the energy furnace and make the entire elaborate event of fitness-building happen more efficiently. Again—consult your physician.

THERE IT IS:
GTF CHROMIUM FOR FITNESS.

CHAPTER 4

WEIGHT

why you gain it, how you lose it, how you keep it off

GLOSSARY

adipose tissue - specialized tissue storing large amounts of fat.

appestat - brain center in hypothalamus controlling appetite.

hormone - substance manufactured in trace amounts in one organ acting as messenger to modulate functions of other tissues or organs.

hypothalamus - part of brain regulating many basic body functions.

insulin resistance - insensitivity of tissue to insulin.

insulin sensitive - ability of cell to receive insulin.

obese - state of having a body weight 20 percent or more above ideal weight for height, sex, and build.

receptor site - receiver on surface of cell which allows cell to combine with substances coursing through blood.

thyroid hormones - hormones produced by thyroid affecting metabolic processes, including glucose absorption and utilization, caloric activity, and metabolism of energy nutrients.

> *T4 (thyroxine)*: thyroid hormone released into blood stream; precursor of T3
>
> *T3 (triidothyronine): active thyroid hormone*

tryptophan - essential amino acid; precursor of serotonin.

serotonin - neurotransmitter; vehicle of communication between nerve cells.

CHROMIUM AS A FAT FIGHTER

There is no such thing as being perfectly healthy but somewhat overweight

---

WEIGHT: WHY YOU GAIN IT

AN UPSCALE TREND (LITERALLY)

Wouldn't you know it—the only place you can be sure of losing weight as you age is in your brain. (You lose about three ounces over the years.[1]) If you're one of the majority of Americans who is overweight, either by just a few pounds or enough to be obese, this chapter should intrigue you. And if it's any solace, you're not alone. The past several decades have seen a steadily increasing proportion of overweight adults in the United States, especially among women.[2] At present, approximately one in five adult Americans, or 34 million people, are obese, as defined by weight that is 20 percent or more above the desirable level.[3] And nine in ten Americans are overweight as defined by their own standards—90 percent *think* they are overweight.

Unfortunately, fat cells are very economical and efficient in energy storage.

CLASSIFICATIONS OF OBESITY

Obesity can be divided into two causative classifications—*hyperplastic*, which refers to increased numbers of fat cells, and *hypertrophic*, which pertains to increased size of fat cells (the same number of cells, just fatter ones). Most people couldn't care less about such details. "Just tell me how to get my weight down, easily, and keep it that way, forevermore. That's all I want to know."

But weight control is complicated with unlimited influences and no easy solutions. Unfortunately, the consequences go beyond the frustrations of having a negative self-image.

WHEN YOU LOSE WEIGHT YOU LOSE MORE THAN FAT: YOU ALSO SURRENDER LEAN BODY MASS.

CORRELATIONS OF OBESITY

Some individuals may be so weight-sensitive they experience negative consequences with relatively small weight gains. On the other hand, others can realize very positive effects from small weight losses.[4]

There is no such thing as being perfectly healthy but somewhat overweight.

Overweight people are more subject to:

»heightened sensitivity to pain

»two to four times the risk for heart disease, high blood pressure, strokes, cancer, and diabetes

»increased health risk during surgery
»more common abdominal hernias
»more frequent degenerative arthritis
»greater incidence of cholesterol gallstones
»lipid (blood fat) abnormalities[5,6,7]

Less serious problems, occurring even in those who are overweight by as little as ten pounds, include: more dandruff, hemorrhoids, flat feet, varicose veins, psychological complaints, dental decay, and slower growth of nails and hair.[8]

NEW KNOWLEDGE FOR AN AGE-OLD PROBLEM

A glut of ongoing research continues to focus on the behavioral and genetic aspects of obesity. Metabolic pathways, however, have not been explored as extensively. These include studies on just when and why and how fat gets deposited in adipose (fat) tissue.

Recently, high technology has helped to uncover a huge mass of new information. For example, enzyme activity can be examined within fat cells—recording changes as they take place in those who are overweight and also during weight loss. This knowledge, previously unknown, is very useful.

We've learned that one enzyme in fat tissue sends a message to your brain to increase caloric intake as soon as weight loss takes place. Thanks a lot! Most of us could do without the zeal of this interfering enzyme to regulate our "fat" affairs. Such control creates another Catch-22 situation, perhaps explaining why we struggle while losing weight, maintaining the urge to overeat. *Too much insulin initiates communication between this enzyme and your brain.*[9]

FAT FACTS
• Blood sugar levels in hungry people are low. • Too much insulin reduces blood sugar levels. • Chromium deprivation creates a chain of events involving impaired insulin metabolism that changes the way your body manages energy and thereby promotes weight gain. • Adjustments during dieting are more complex than a simple wearing down of fat; other metabolic weight-controlling systems are also affected.

Let's see how this knowledge comes together.

THE INSULIN CONNECTION

Recall that insulin plays a major role in energy production. Insulin metabolism affects weight control.

INSULIN HELPS TO:
• reduce appetite • curb sugar and carbohydrate cravings • enhance your capacity to burn calories • manufacture human protein from amino acids

Overall, regulated insulin function increases the availability of glucose and decreases that of fat.[10]

Without chromium, however, insulin's powerful fat-fighting properties may be futile. You learned how chromium is essential for insulin performance and that chromium is in short supply in the American diet. To review, the main reasons for chromium's scarcity are excessive chromium losses caused by: food processing, inadequate dietary supply, refined sugar and other simple carbohydrates in the diet, exercise, and/or your body's inability to convert chromium to its biologically active GTF form.

INSULIN RESISTANCE

Receptor sites are receivers on the surfaces of cells that allow cells to combine with materials travelling through your blood. Insulin receptors are like magnets—they attract insulin, and pull it into your cells.

For reasons not completely understood, your cells sometimes put up a barrier, and refuse to pick up the insulin they require. As explained in Chapter 3, this phenomenon is called *insulin resistance*. According to a study reported in the *American Journal of Clinical Nutrition* on food intake and body weight, this reaction is particularly true of muscle, liver, brain and *adipose* tissue.[11]

You can't really separate the effect of insulin resistance on each of these organs and tissues, because one outcome spawns another. Insulin-resistant muscle and liver both reduce energy reserves. Inertia is the result. As for your brain, when it refuses to admit insulin, thinking capacity suffers. And adipose tissue? Here comes the overweight component. What a triad! Now you're lethargic, dull, *and* overweight. And each of these consequences impacts on the others.

Insulin resistance occurs when there is a defect in either insulin receptor sites or any metabolic function involved in the efficiency of these receptors.[12]

Insulin resistance is a very well known occurrence among those who are overweight.[13] Its consequences have been reported in the medical journals only recently.[14] The "Keep Out" sign posted by your cells causes the insulin level in your blood to rise. High insulin levels can eventually lead to heart disease and diabetes. Last year, a chilling article in the *New England Journal of Medicine* was headlined, "Insulin Resistance: A Secret Killer?"[15]

The relationship between obesity and diabetes has been observed for many years. Although increased weight may be part of the diabetic syndrome, it often serves as a primary factor, actually inducing abnormalities in sugar metabolism and insulin secretion. So it can be both *cause* and *effect*.[16]

To add insult to injury, insulin resistance is responsible for excess glucose remaining in your blood. Some of this glucose may be converted to precursors of fats called *triglycerides*, which eventually become incorporated into fatty tissue. What you don't need now is more fat tissue.

APPETITE CONTROL: THE HYPOTHALAMUS APPESTAT

Lying near the underside of your brain, just about in the center of your head, is your hypothalamus (Greek for *under the inner room*). Not much bigger than a small prune, this incredible, but seemingly trivial, mass of cells acts as the command post for your brain. It's the message center that maintains equilibrium and informs other regions of your brain of their duties.

A portion of your hypothalamus is called the *satiety* center, or *appestat*. The appestat controls your appetite by communicating with your brain.[17] Did you know that you don't have the sensation of hunger until your hypothalamus sends a hunger signal to your brain? Falling blood sugar and a mild sensation of fatigue prompt this hunger indicator, setting a chain of events in motion.

Low blood sugar causes:

»your hypothalamus to send impulses to step up production of gastric juices and saliva;
»your stomach to increase the speed and force of its contractions;
»your taste buds to become more sensitive.

THE FINAL DEMAND IS: FEED ME! NOW!

Insulin has a precipitous and profound effect on your appetite-regulating gland. As you eat and your blood glucose level rises, your pancreas secretes insulin to take care of the newly arrived glucose. And as your insulin level increases, your appestat is affected, and your hunger is satisfied.[18,19]

A similar outcome has been demonstrated by the uptake of insulin directly into your cerebrospinal fluid, and subsequently into your brain. (Cerebrospinal fluid fills the cavity inside the vertebrate brain and spinal cord.) Stimulation of insulin receptors in your brain also causes a reduction of food intake.[20,21]

YOUR APPESTAT IS RESPONSIVE TO INSULIN LEVELS, NOT TO THE QUANTITY OF FOOD INTAKE.

These are wonderful blueprints for control—if only they functioned with efficiency all the time. Here's the rub: insulin resistance prevents this mechanism from working and leads to a false perception of the inadequacy of food, resulting in overeating.[22] You may have plenty of insulin, but if your cell receptors can't recognize and utilize any of it, you just go on packing it away. (And all this time you thought you were "pigging out" because of lack of will power! Isn't it reassuring to know that's not the case?)

These maneuvers of appetite communication malfunction in different ways. If one control mechanism is impaired, you eat more than you need to. If the other is down, you don't consume enough. When you lose the right oar while rowing, the boat turns one way. You lose the left oar, and the boat swings the other way. And so it is when these feedback systems are thrown off balance.

SUGAR CRAVINGS AND SEROTONIN PRODUCTION

When the behavior-regulating neurotransmitter, *serotonin,* is out of order, it has been shown to cause uncurbed binge-eating. The result is excessive consumption of refined carbohydrates, and/or cravings for sweets.[23,24]

Serotonin is made in your brain from tryptophan, an essential amino acid present in most foods. But tryptophan needs insulin to get into your brain.[25,26] Normally, a high carbohydrate meal stimulates insulin secretion, which enhances tryptophan uptake by your brain. But when insulin metabolism is not working properly, up goes another "Do-Not-Enter" sign; tryptophan has no way of getting through, and serotonin production breaks down. Without serotonin, the message to suppress the urge for carbohydrates is never given. Instead of *curbing*, you experience *craving*—your desire to eat continues. And now you have a biological and scientific excuse for excessive consumption of ice cream (or maybe it's chocolate cake; mine is pecan pie).

CARBOHYDRATE CRAVINGS CAN REPRESENT A DEFICIENCY OF SEROTONIN RATHER THAN A NEED FOR FOOD.[27]

To summarize this progression of events:
»insulin resistance puts up road blocks against tryptophan absorption into your brain
»which suppresses serotonin production
»which leads to binge-eating
»which leads to chromium depletion
»which leads to increased insulin resistance

And so the tryptophan embargo and serotonin inadequacy continue. Impaired serotonin metabolism is at the end of a chain of events initiated with insulin resistance. A vicious cycle is under way. (*There's a hole in the bucket, Dear Liza, Dear Liza.*)

THYROID IMPAIRMENT

Remember the old excuse for overweight? Anyone with extra pounds had a "glandular" disorder. That theory became outdated and was replaced by discussions of set point, will power, behavior modification, exercise, and/or energy expenditure. Guess what? Things have come full cycle, and we are back to glandular again. The fact is that unbalanced glandular status, particularly of the thyroid, can contribute to chronic, recalcitrant obesity.

You now have the picture of a very complex biochemistry involved in weight management. Blood glucose, thyroid hormones, appestat, and fat cell enzymes do not have a monopoly on food-control minipulation. You can see that these processes cause the body to get fatter and fatter while you remain hungry, weak, and inactive, and couch-potato status is achieved.

Do you need to be a graduate biochemist to understand all the controls for weight management? No! But a little knowledge can be helpful. GTF chromium, by helping to normalize most of these functions and by assisting in balancing insulin metabolism, has contributed to a changing way of thinking about the causes for overweight.

WEIGHT: HOW YOU LOSE IT

WEIGHT LOSS AND CHROMIUM SUPPLEMENTATION

I discovered in my own personal laboratory (me!) that chromium supplementaion affects food intake. This fact is confirmed by many scientific reports, including one cited recently in the *American Journal of Clinical Nutrition.*[28] The addition of GTF chromium has a dramatic effect on my intimate responses to low blood sugar, and to my weight. Yes, chromium can be a dietary counterpart in the reduction and control of body weight.

George Boucher is a Nebraska cattle rancher. His goal is to persuade farmers and ranchers to stop the use of synthetic fertilizers and crop spraying. Boucher is in constant search of supplements to keep his livestock free of disease. "I am continually looking for methods to supply the healthiest meat to the meat-eating public—ways to compensate for the herbicides and pesticides that are so solidly entrenched in our culture," said Boucher.

Boucher read about the health benefits of chromium polynicotinate, and added this trace mineral to the daily feed for his lambs. He checked the results against another group—animals receiving the same diet, but without the addition of chromium. For Mr. Boucher, this experiment was a dim failure from a marketing point of view, but for those who want to lose weight, the experiment offers exciting hope: *the animals receiving the chromium ate more food, had reduced fat, weighed a couple of pounds less, and had more lean body mass!*

The chromium-fed lambs also exhibited more energy, and less lethargy in mid-day heat. Mr. Boucher was surprised that not a single lamb had "wet eye" or "runny nose." The wool on these animals looked particularly healthy. Although Mr. Boucher appreciated the fine appearance of the carcasses, he lost out financially because these animals did not come up to "grade" for the marketplace: they did not weigh in at the required 116 pounds because of lack of fat.

The significant aspect is that the chromium-fed lambs did not have the fat cover usually seen in top-graded animals. They had six-and-a-half pounds of additional lean body mass, and less fat.

Boucher continued his experiment with knife and fork. He reported that the lamb meat was spectacular—it was tender and lean. Isn't it an irony that the consumer pays premium prices for fat-laden meat (considered the quality standard), yet the Surgeon General tells us to cut away any visible fat—with further instructions to let fat drippings go down the drain, rather than into our stomachs?[29]

From our point of view, the success of Boucher's experiments indicate that victory in coping with weight problems may be a chromium supplement away.

OVERCOMING INSULIN RESISTANCE

Sometimes your adipose tissue can easily gobble up excess insulin (the cells are insulin sensitive), available only because your muscles put out the "No Vacancy" sign (now the cells are insulin resistant). Restoring the insulin sensitivity of your muscles returns insulin levels to normal, thus removing a stimulus for obesity.[30,31]

Chromium therapy for obese individuals is at the beginning stages of controlled clinical studies, but it is already widely in use by grass roots America. The results so far are very promising. We looked at several cases of successful chromium therapy used to overcome insulin resistance, including a few reported in the *Journal of the American Medical Association*.[32] These studies suggest that one explanation for insulin resistance is a deprivation of biologically active GTF chromium![33] Chromium enables insulin to cross the barrier.

COMPELLING SCIENTIFIC AFFIRMATION
AND AN ABUNDANCE OF
CLINICAL EXPERIENCE RELATE
CHROMIUM AND WEIGHT LOSS.

EFFECT OF INSULIN ON YOUR HYPOTHALAMUS

How does the hypothalamus regulate appetite control? We know that glucose deprivation increases food intake. We also know that carbohydrates lead to more blood-sugar stability than either fat or protein. So it has been postulated that there are sensitive receptors in the nuclei of the hypothalamus which respond to glucose.[34]

Enter GTF chromium, which helps to overcome insulin resistance and/or enhance insulin action, allowing for a faster, fuller expression of the satiety signal by helping to bring glucose into your cells.

SUGAR CURBING AND SEROTONIN PRODUCTION

The unkind cycle of serotonin blockage is broken by the improvement of insulin action with the use of GTF chromium.

Now the equation changes:
»chromium leads to insulin sensitivity
»which leads to tryptophan entry
»which leads to serotonin production
»which leads to *controlled* eating

NUTRIENTS AND DRUGS KNOWN TO ENHANCE THE PRODUCTION OR THE ACTION OF SEROTONIN ARE CURRENTLY BEING TESTED AS TREATMENTS FOR CARBOHYDRATE CRAVING. BECAUSE OBSESSIVE/COMPULSIVE DISORDERS IN GENERAL MAY BE DUE TO A RELATIVE LACK OF SEROTONIN, THEY, TOO, ARE BEING EXAMINED.[35,36]

FAT-BURNING:
IMPROVING FUNCTIONAL THYROID STATUS

Thyroid hormones control your body's basal metabolism—the resting rate at which you burn calories for energy. These hormones also increase the mobilization and burning of fat reserves for energy—just what you want. Thyroid hormones divert calories away from storage as fat, so that they get used up as energy.[37] Physicians practicing at the time of Hippocrates recommended that overweight people eat while they were still panting, just after exercise. They must have known about increased metabolic rate!

As in many cascading processes, one thyroid hormone is a catalyst for another. Thyroxine (T4), the thyroid hormone released into your blood stream, is converted to triidothyronine (T3)—the active thyroid hormone. T3 is the hormone that produces the fat "round-up."

It is well established that carbohydrates stimulate the conversion of T4 to T3. If you are on a low-calorie or low-complex-carbohydrate diet, the conversion is depressed. It also slumps in the uncontrolled, insulin-dependent diabetic, but can be reversed with insulin therapy. These facts indicate that it isn't the carbohydrates per se that stimulate T4/T3 conversion, but the insulin secreted by your pancreas, and, again, this is activated by complex carbohydrate consumption. Similar research has been reported in the last decade in *Annals of Review of Medicine*, *Metabolism*, and the *International Journal of Obesity*.[38,39,40]

In summary, insulin-resistant overweight people may suffer from depressed T4/T3 conversion, which is exacerbated by low-calorie, low complex-carbohydrate diets.

You can see how a low-calorie diet can work against you. Enhancement of insulin action with GTF chromium may help to maintain normal T4/T3 conversion, even if you are dieting and/or you are not getting enough calories or carbohydrates.

WEIGHT: HOW YOU KEEP IT OFF

PREVENTING THE REBOUND EFFECT TO MAINTAIN MUSCLE MASS

Many people start dieting and almost immediately lose weight. It has been said that weight clinics succeed on their failure. You visit the fat-reducing salon, you lose weight, you gain weight, and you return to the salon. Another "hole-in-the-bucket."

Soon, problems are encountered because weight is lost by reducing both fat and protein. It gets harder and harder to lose weight. Lack of insulin (the result of a low calorie diet), actually causes a breakdown of muscle tissue. More than half the weight lost while dieting may be lean muscle tissue, thereby impairing your ability to keep the weight off.

Muscles use more calories than fat. So loss of muscle tissue reduces your body's calorie-burning capacity. Example: you may start out with a calorie-burning rate of 70 calories per hour. After losing weight, this rate may drop down to 50 calories an hour. Since your ability to burn calories is now reduced, it is much more difficult to keep the weight off—one reason why many people find it tougher to maintain their lower weight than it was to lose the weight in the first place. Gaining weight in less time than it took to lose it is called the *rebound effect*—an almost inevitable consequence for those who diet on low-carbohydrate regimens.

WITH THE LOSS OF LEAN MASS
YOU MAINTAIN AND GAIN WEIGHT
ON FEWER CALORIES.

To add to the problem, muscle tissue of the overweight is often insulin-resistant.[41]

You can see why dieters lose lean muscle mass as fast or faster than they lose fat. Recall from Chapter 3 that insulin is anti-catabolic: it strongly inhibits the breakdown of body proteins. Because of its influence on insulin, chromium can slow the loss of lean body mass. It can maintain the metabolic rate to dampen the rebound phenomenon, and reduce insulin resistance.

In summary, the strategy is to spare lean muscle mass while dieting, and to help maintain your metabolic rate for the future—to assist you during your post-diet maintenance phase. GTF chromium, by enhancing the anabolic action of insulin on muscle, helps to build and maintain more of your chief calorie-burning tissues.

FOOD CHOICES TO REDUCE HUNGER

Your digestive system is admirably designed to be the ultimate food processor. Food is broken down in nice, orderly, nature-designed fashion, so that eventually it becomes your energy supply. But when you swallow foods that the manufacturer or the Cuisenart has taken apart for you, your cells respond in strange ways.

One of the most exciting and important food studies ever conducted was reported in 1977 in Britain's prestigious medical journal, *Lancet.* Amounts of apples and apple juice, equal in calories, were fed to two groups of people. After consumption, blood glucose was measured, and found to have increased equally in both groups. But the levels fell during the second and third hours only in the juice group! Your insulin control panel reads glucose differently, depending on its source: its reply to apple juice is 50 percent greater than it is to apples, even though calorie consumption is identical.

Even more fascinating: responses of a third group of people who consumed an equal caloric amount of apple sauce, showed results in between those of the whole fruit and the juice. The only difference between the whole apple and the apple sauce was that the apple was puréed. Nothing was added, nothing taken away. But responses vary when texture is different. Your body handles food differently if you don't have to chew, even though the fiber and caloric content are the same. Since this report first appeared, many similar studies have been conducted. The same disparities are found between oranges and orange juice, and so on.

Greater insulin production caused by liquid food (fruit juices) represents the reaction of your pancreas to more rapid absorption of fiber-free, simple carbohydrate. And now you know the rest of the story:

»juices (instead of intact food) create too much insulin
»too much insulin gobbles up blood glucose
»which stimulates appetite

THE REBOUND FALL IN BLOOD GLUCOSE THAT FOLLOWS THE CONSUMPTION OF FRUIT JUICES AND OTHER SUGARY DRINKS *PROMOTES OBESITY* BY ENCOURAGING AN EARLIER RESUMPTION OF EATING.[42]

So an extremely important technique for keeping weight off is to consume *intact food* exclusively: a whole apple instead of apple sauce; carrots instead of carrot salad. Since this is unrealistic for most of us all the time, GTF chromium should help to mitigate the rebound fall.

THE EXERCISE CONNECTION

We've heard it a million times (literally!). The fat in your diet and your level of activity are the major determinants of obesity. How many blocks you walk, stairs you climb, and sports you participate in play a major role. But this explains only part of the problem. The interrelations of body movement and fat deposits are extremely complex. The degree of your physical activity is an important factor of glucose intolerance.[43]

Here's a serendipitous cycle:

»exercise improves the sensitivity of receptor sites
»which allows insulin to be properly activated
»which allows glucose to convert to glycogen
»which helps to maintain normal levels of glucose in your blood
»which helps to prevent hunger and to increase your energy stores
»which gives you pep, power, and punch to exercise

Strategies for getting started on an exercise program are outlined in Chapter 8.

CONCLUSION

The reason I was inspired to do research on chromium is because GTF chromium polynicotinate supplementation has worked for me and my family, and for the patients of the physicians with whom I interact.

Those who are overweight are at special risk for chromium deficiency. You can begin to understand why the discovery of the significance of GTF chromium by Dr. Walter Mertz has been embraced as one of the most outstanding disclosures of the mid-twentieth century. Sure, we have computers, data bases, telephones, radios, TV, air travel, satellites, and the printed word (including the ability to drop leaflets from the sky). It still takes many years from the time a discovery is recognized to the time the significance of that revelation is applied—no matter how stunning or health-promoting that science may be.

Some researchers believe that supplementing with chromium causes weight loss because it potentiates insulin utilization, thereby reducing an overabundance of circulating levels of insulin; others believe that the weight loss may also result from a mild appetite-reducing effect of the chromium itself.[44] While the researchers debate about the precise metabolic pathways involved, most of us say, "We don't care how it works. We care that it does work."

Changing people's behavior is not easy. But even modest reductions in weight have a marked effect on well being and on health risk.[45] We know that GTF chromium may, at the very least, be responsible for the loss of a few pounds.

THE ONLY WAY YOU CAN MASTER NATURE
IS TO COOPERATE WITH IT,
AND ABIDE BY ITS BIDDING.

CASE HISTORY

Dr. Michael Rosenbaum, of Corte Madera, California, has been aware of the effect of chromium supplementation on sugar craving since 1977. Recently, Jane, a patient who consumed sweets all her life, called, in tears. "I've been doing so well for three weeks on your program, Dr. Rosenbaum," she cried. "But two days ago, I lost it, and I've been stuffing myself like crazy ever since."

Dr. Rosenbaum looked at Jane's chart. "I see that you started taking chromium supplements just about three weeks ago." Jane interrupted with a shriek. "Oh, my goodness! I've been out of chromium for four days. The binge-eating started two days ago. Do you think—?"

Dr. Rosenbaum more than "thought." He knew! The doctor repeated the information he had imparted to Jane initially. He explained again how chromium affects sugar metabolism, which in turn affects cravings. The fact that Jane didn't make the connection between the cravings and chromium deficiency eliminated the possibility of the placebo effect. Dr. Rosenbaum reports that 50 percent of his patients with eating disorders respond very well to chromium polynicotinate supplementation, 30 percent respond partially, and 10 to 20 percent have no success. (The failures occur because disorders are caused by factors other than chromium deficiencies—such as food allergy, etc.)

Sally, another patient, chided Dr. Rosenbaum for prescribing chromium polynicotinate because her bread and croissant cravings had all but vanished. Although she pretended to feel deprived, she was happily losing weight.[46]

THERE IT IS: GTF CHROMIUM FOR WEIGHT CONTROL

CHAPTER **5**

STRESS

what it is, how you cope with it

GLOSSARY

adrenalin - also called epinephrine; serves as counterregulatory function to break down liver and muscle glycogen; especially useful mode of action in times of stress.

adaptation - adjustment of organism in response to adverse stimulus; necessary for survival.

arousal mechanism - alarm "bell" turning on fight-or-flight response.

autonomic mechanism - reaction functioning without conscious effort.

fight-or-flight response - reaction triggered by confrontation with stressor.

stress - nonspecific response to any demand.

CHROMIUM AS A STRESS RESISTOR

If your stress mechanisms are well nourished, they won't break down.

STRESS: WHAT IT IS

"EAT SOMETHING"

I had three children (four, counting our niece who came to live with us at age nine), a large house, a growing business, one or two important hobbies, and a few other "extended-family" obligations. I could handle it—most of the time. When I did lose control, my husband would say, "Eat something."

This infuriated me! I was wildly upset, and he told me to eat. But my astute husband had noticed that regardless of the reason for my stress, or the level of my agony, I calmed down after eating. Little did I realize that *what* I ate and *when* I ate caused me to lose control or over-react to minor situations.

STRESS REACTIONS

What provokes stress in *your* life? Is it talking to your mother-in-law, who is constantly telling you what to do? What makes you anxious? Is it waiting for a friend or business associate, who is late for your limited-time appointment? And how do you react under these circumstances? Do your reactions vary at different times of the day?

At least 1400 bio-physical responses are noted to be caused by stress and anxiety.

STRESS RESPONSES	
• lightheadedness	• perceptual changes
• dizziness	• rubbery legs
• tingling sensations	• impotence
• restlessness	• stomach fluttering
• dry mouth	• throat tightness
• lack of energy	• diarrhea
• constipation	• insomnia
• nightmares	• noise sensitivity
• back pains	• overeating
• frequent urination	• irritability
• depression	• fatigue

Can you identify with any of the listed responses? Chances are you can add to the list.

THE ARRAY OF SYMPTOMS CHARACTERIZING STRESS OR ANXIETY ARE SO CONFUSING AND SO NUMEROUS THAT ACCURATE DIAGNOSIS IS OFTEN DIFFICULT.

You may be attacked at your weak points—your head, your stomach, your back. Stress can affect an organ that is not quite up to par, particularly one that plays a role in stress management, such as your hypothalamus. Or, like me (the old me), it could be an emotional response.

DEFINING STRESS

What is stress, anyway? Stress is a private event, a direct consequence of how you define your personal relationship to the world. It doesn't matter whether or not a stressful situation actually exists. The precipitating factor is your decision that some kind of threat—emotional or physical—is present.[1]

STRESS IS TRADITIONALLY DEFINED AS THE ACTIVATION OF THE AROUSAL MECHANISM—THE ALARM AGENT DESCRIBED AS FIGHT-OR-FLIGHT.

When the signal is set off, the stress reaction begins at the level of your midbrain. The image of an uncomfortable situation travels from your cortex (the outer layer of gray matter in your brain which receives sensory stimuli) to your brain's deeper structures.

One of the most important of these deep structures is your hypothalamus, which is top kingpin of your brain's relay setup. It works like a dispatching station of a telecommunications center—its call of warning ready to dart out at a microsecond's notice.

Once your uneasy status has been sensed, your hypothalamus radiates stimulating impulses to its entire territory, alerting all of you to the circumstances of the threatening world outside. That's the stress effect. All of you reacts, and does so with the speed of an electronic messenger. And you respond in any or several of those 1400 possible ways. These reactions have protected humans over a million years of time, whether faced with a wild animal about to attack or with the wild idea of asking your boss for a raise. You may be a twenty-first-century person, but you respond to stress with pre-history biochemistry. Whether sparked by threats of survival or emotional upheavals, your response is similar.

One of the reactions which follows is the production of adrenalin (now called epinephrine), the release of which is mainly sensitive to conditions of stress. How many times have you heard or used the expression, "I could feel my adrenalin flowing," or, "I was stoked up," expressions denoting excitation.

But that's just the tip of the iceberg. The might of your hypothalamus puts the seventeenth-century British Empire to shame. Your hypothalamus is in command of activating, empowering, and integrating your autonomic mechanisms—those which get turned on without conscious effort. These include endocrine activities—the ones responsible for hormonal secretions, fluid regulation, body temperature control, sleep patterns, and basic drives such as hunger, and even sex.

Additionally, your pituitary, considered a master gland because it regulates the release of hormones from other glands, is *under the bidding of your hypothalamus.* A special set of blood vessels connects your pituitary and your hypothalamus, carrying messages from one to the other. Chemicals released by your hypothalamus zip over the half-inch distance to your pituitary and commission it to go into action.

When hormones from other glands reach high levels in your bloodstream, they send a message to your hypothalamus to cease and desist—to stop releasing additional chemicals. Your hypothalamus has been considered as the possible primary site triggering the onset of aging at all levels of your being.[2] And, as you already know, insulin plays a major role.

INSULIN HAS A PROFOUND EFFECT ON YOUR HYPOTHALAMUS.

AUTOMATIC STRESS REACTIONS

Of special concern when under stress are the functions that occur automatically in the large organs of your body—contractions of your heart and your spleen, the movement of your gut, the secretion of digestive enzymes, the processes of perspiring and blood coagulation, dilation of your pupils—to name a few.

Suppose you're at the top of a roller coaster. Or perhaps in an elevator, on the highest floor. Suddenly, you come to a halt. A siren sounds. Someone bellows: "It's broken." Your heart beats faster—raising your blood pressure,. You increase oxygen-carrying capacity, breathe more deeply, and more blood is redirected to your brain and muscles. Your entire body snaps into its fight-or-flight mode, even though you can do neither at the moment. Your hypothalamus is responsible for generating this all-out cascade of events.

You can feel some of the consequences—racing heart, churning stomach, dry mouth, trembling hands. But you are unaware of your body's delivery of glucose, stored as glycogen in your liver, as you answer to the stress situation.[3]

STORED ENERGY: THE STRESS BUFFER

Little doubt exists that a broad range of hormones respond to stress. Catabolic hormone levels increase; anabolic levels are suppressed. In stress-producing situations, glucose is your most important source of immediately available energy. Both your central nervous system and musculature are almost entirely dependent on glucose for their efficient performance. Neuromuscular activity is critical in permitting and controlling your behavioral responses to stress.

Glucose is also required as a source of energy for the repair and regeneration of tissues which have been damaged during the execution of stress responses. In contrast to fats and proteins (the other possible sources of energy), carbohydrates do not tend to yield toxic metabolites, even when large quantities are suddenly broken down. Utilization of glucose proceeds without risk even if stress is so severe that it disrupts liver detoxification or elimination processes. (Diarrhea and constipation can be reactions to stress.)

IN ACUTE EMERGENCIES, YOU ARE DEPENDENT ON YOUR CARBOHYDRATE RESERVES, AND PRIMARILY ON BLOOD GLUCOSE.

STRESS IS NON-SPECIFIC

Hans Selye was the first to say that stress was nonspecific. Regardless of the reason for stress (physical, chemical, or emotional), your response may be the same: it is not explicit to the cause. (It doesn't matter, for example, if you have no money because you are out of work, lost it all in a game of poker, or gave it away in alimony payments—the physical consequences of the stress of being broke are identical.)

Selye also proposed that stress may be the villain in many degenerative diseases as well as a cause for abnormalities. He was ahead of his time by at least half a century. His concept was indeed wholistic.

Since we know that your brain is involved in stress reactions—and we even understand some of the mechanisms—the chain of events which lead to the pathology of stress can be broken. And that's the rationale for using nutrition to deal with stress. *You can alter the level of physical experience.* Nutrients, like tools, are a means to an end.

IF YOUR STRESS MECHANISMS ARE WELL NOURISHED, THEY WILL NOT BREAK DOWN. YOU CAN HELP TO PREVENT STRESS DAMAGE.

STRESS: HOW TO COPE WITH IT

THE IDEAL CONTROL SYSTEM

You've learned from earlier chapters that the concentration of glucose in your blood is kept within range by a complex set of regulatory mechanisms. This management system works especially well if:

»you eat several small complex carbohydrate meals during the day, instead of three larger meals

»these smaller meals contain all the nutrients required for glucose metabolism

»you avoid all simple, refined carbohydrates, which deplete chromium stores.

Such a regime not only buffers stress, but also keeps weight under control, helps to protect your heart, and provides more energy. But this is not a way of life for most of us. Few people abide by—or find it comfortable or even *possible* to—follow these tenets every day in every way. Knowledge, however, is the beginning of change.

What happens when large quantities of food are consumed at a single meal? Your blood glucose level rises dramatically. As explained earlier, your body tissues interpret high blood glucose as bad news, and so they swing into action, mobilizing all the defense mechanisms at their disposal.

WHEN YOU EAT TOO MUCH AT A MEAL
• The first line of defense occurs when much of that glucose is converted to glycogen and stored for later use • The second line of defense is provided by various endocrine secretions which also affect your blood sugar level

Insulin is an extremely important hormone affecting your blood sugar level. As you know, insulin is a protein released by your pancreas. It lowers blood glucose levels, and accomplishes this important mission in two ways:

»It stimulates your liver to convert glucose to glycogen.
»It facilitates passage of glucose from your blood into body cells.

The output of insulin is directly controlled by the level of glucose in your blood. This mechanism provides a good example of a negative-feedback, closed-loop control system, similar to that of an automatic air conditioning unit: the warm air in a room turns on the air conditioner; when the air falls under the action of the air conditioner and cools down, the air conditioner shuts off. When glucose rises after a meal, more insulin is released; as the glucose falls under the action of insulin, the insulin-producing mechanism is turned off.

Although a few other pathways control insulin output, direct command by blood glucose levels appears to be the most important for moment-to-moment control. Recall that in the absence of insulin, many cells are virtually impermeable to glucose.

ADRENALIN AND GLUCOSE REGULATION IN EMERGENCIES

To understand glucose regulation at times of stress, several points need to be clear. You already know that glucose is stored as glycogen in liver and in muscle, and that when under stress there is a call on glucose to provide you with energy. Under these circumstances, blood glucose may be insufficient, so stored glucose must be released. But glycogen is held captive as a complex matrix. Adrenalin, released under stress, acts on glycogen just as a microwave defrosts frozen food more quickly.

ADRENALIN HASTENS THE CONVERSION OF GLYCOGEN TO GLUCOSE, A CATABOLIC RESPONSE.

Although not routinely important in the control of blood glucose, adrenalin is, therefore, of great significance in emergencies because it raises blood glucose levels rapidly. It does this not only by stimulating the breakdown of glycogen to glucose, but also by slowing down the rate at which muscle cells pick up glucose from your blood.

Muscle cells, which need the glucose and which contain some glycogen, face no problem. Neither do brain cells, which do not require insulin to promote their supply of glucose. It's interesting to note that other body cells containing glucose are controlled by agents which now inhibit its release. This insures that the brain and muscle get the supply of glucose.

Brain cells, because they do not store glucose or require insulin to accept it, are directly and uniquely reliant on circulating blood glucose. Typical of so many body pathways involving the brain, these cells are given priority. This is good news and bad news. It's great that glucose is immediately available for your brain. But if your blood glucose is low, you experience all the symptoms of hypoglycemia involving emotion: panic, fear, inability to cope, and so on.

Research done in 1968 and 1975 shows how blood glucose responds to recovery from stress.[4,5] On the removal of stress, the levels fall back to and perhaps below normal, as part of a pattern of anabolic response. It's not just that the breakdown period has stopped, but the decrease in blood glucose levels also involves an active anabolic (building up) process.

IN AN ATTEMPT TO REPLACE THE GLUCOSE LOST TO YOUR LIVER AND MUSCLES WHEN YOU EXPERIENCE STRESS, YOUR BLOOD GLUCOSE DECLINES.

ANNOYING OR SUSTAINED STRESS

To complicate the issue, it has also been shown that sustained stress lowers blood glucose. This refers to stress that is more of an ongoing annoyance—irritants such as a constant noise or a nagging child, experiences which elicit a different response from that of a more threatening hazard. The initial rise in blood sugar causes the pancreas to overreact, and the abundant insulin lowers your blood sugar.

ONE OF THE MOST FREQUENT ACTIVATORS OF HYPOGLYCEMIA IS AN ONGOING NUISANCE DISTURBANCE.

If the duration of stress is extended, the efficiency of the adrenals will be impaired, and so hypoglycemia is prolonged. On recovery, however, blood glucose usually returns to normal.[6]

BLOOD SUGAR AND THE BLUES

You have seen how stress affects your blood sugar. Can blood sugar affect your stress level? Can you feel stressed simply because your blood sugar levels are low? The answer is definitely *yes*!

Because of insulin's involvement with blood sugar, it is correlated with the highs and lows that make you feel tired and irritable, or alive and full of energy. You know that when insulin "pumps" glucose inside your cells, you feel "up" because glucose is used for energy. When blood sugar is low, energy is reduced, resulting in feelings of lethargy, sluggishness, and the "blues." Severe or chronic low blood sugar can be responsible for more severe symptoms of anxiety, depression, irritability, and insomnia.

High blood sugar (hyperglycemia) causes problems which include drowsiness, weakness, and fatigue.[7] In either case, your stress syndrome is aggravated. (More on hyperglycemia in Chapter 7.)

SEROTONIN, TRYPTOPHAN AND STRESS

At least a dozen studies have shown that serotonin precursors improve mood disorders. As explained, serotonin is the chemical messenger which transmits impulses between brain cells. Tryptophan, a very important amino acid, is a significant precursor of serotonin. (A precursor precedes and is the source of another substance.)

Tryptophan's tranquilizing and sleep-inducing effects are well documented in scientific literature. Again, its role in stress physiology relates to its requirement for the manufacture of serotonin, the actual neurotransmitter involved in promoting sleep and relaxation.

But tryptophan is unable to enter your brain without insulin.

BY ENHANCING INSULIN ACTION,
CHROMIUM HELPS TO INCREASE
TRYPTOPHAN UPTAKE
AND SEROTONIN SYNTHESIS,
PROMOTING SLEEP AND RELAXATION.

COMPLEX CARBOHYDRATES AND TRYPTOPHAN

Here's another plus for the complex carbohydrate regimen: a high-protein meal retards the uptake of tryptophan into your brain. This happens because such a meal increases the concentrations of other amino acids that compete with the tryptophan. The higher the protein content of a particular meal, the more difficult it is for tryptophan to enter your brain. Carbohydrate, by stimulating insulin secretion, lowers the blood concentration of the competing amino acids, thereby increasing the tryptophan/amino acid ratio.[8]

ALTERING YOUR STRESS RESPONSE

It's not difficult to get advice about altering the way in which you cope with stress on an emotional level. Books, classes, radio talk shows, magazine articles, even rap sessions in your exercise class, abound with such information. Changing your biophysical response is another matter. Despite the fact that these reactions can be modified, which in turn changes behavioral reactions, this aspect has been ignored almost entirely by stress researchers.[9] Only a handful of experiments have been done on the subject to date.

A report in the *Journal of International Research Communications* shows that increasing carbohydrates just before exposure to low levels of stress (in the form of noise) improved worker's performance.[10] Another study, cited in *Proceedings of the Nutrition Society,* demonstrated that high accident rates in an iron foundry in England were associated with low carbohydrate intake,[11] and that the converse was true: there were low accident rates with high carbohydrate intake.[12] High carbohydrate intake produces a relative elevation, or normalization, of blood glucose levels, offering some protection from the effects of stress.

It has also been observed that blood glucose levels of automobile crash victims are surprisingly low.

THE NIACIN CONNECTION

Niacin deficiency has been related to depression and anxiety. One theory is that when there is a niacin deficiency, tryptophan is utilized to produce this important B-complex nutrient. So now there is less tryptophan available for the production of serotonin. *Low serotonin has been associated with depression.*[13]

Research reported in *Society, Stress, and Disease*, indicates that the elevation of the blood level of free fatty acids can be blocked by prior administration of nicotinic acid.[14]

RAISED FREE FATTY ACIDS ARE PART OF THE PATTERN OF PHYSIOLOGICAL STRESS.

GTF chromium polynicotinate contains a few molecules of niacin. So here are two more reasons for favoring niacin-bound GTF supplementation (*chromium polynicotinate*).

Subclinical pellagra, a disease that symptomatically mimics schizophrenia, has been shown to be relieved with small quantities of niacin.[15] Some schizophrenics respond to extra niacin and many have impaired glucose tolerance.

What are the possibilities of related therapy for other psychological problems? Are other types of mental disorder produced by deficiencies of GTF chromium? Would large doses of niacin make our trivial dietary amounts of chromium more effective? Hopefully, we'll have the answers from the researchers soon.

CHROMIUM DEFICIENCY AND STRESS

Under extreme stress, urinary chromium excretion can be as much as fifty-fold. This loss can continue for several days.

THE EFFECTS OF CHROMIUM DEFICIENCY ARE MORE INTENSE WHEN YOU ARE UNDER STRESS.

An interesting study demonstrated that the negative effects of chromium deficiency are exacerbated when subjected to stress. One reaction mimics that of insulin deficiency.[16] The fact that glycogen is released from your liver when you are under stress helps to clarify this phenomenon.

At the risk of sounding like a broken record:

»Chromium potentiates insulin
»which in turn helps to overcome insulin resistance
»which in turn helps to optimize the function of your hypothalamus

The use of biologically active niacin-bound GTF chromium as a nutritional adjunct in stress control is based on its ability to overcome insulin resistance and/or to enhance the effects of insulin—which in turn normalizes glucose function.

SUMMARY

Stress increases energy requirements and creates a demand for an expanded supply of energy-yielding glucose. Once again we see the chromium/insulin dependency. Wouldn't it be wonderful if emotions such as anger, anxiety, depression, fear, grief, guilt, jealousy and shame—emotions associated with stress—could be tempered simply by controlling blood sugar levels? GTF chromium polynicotinate may be able to do just that in some circumstances.

Sadly, a whole generation of medical doctors and scientists in this country appear to be unaware that stress and anxiety can be diminished with attempts to normalize metabolic pathways.

TAKING DRUGS TO REDUCE THE
DELETERIOUS EFFECTS OF STRESS
IS LIKE MOPPING THE FLOOR WHEN
THE SINK IS OVERFLOWING
INSTEAD OF TURNING OFF THE FAUCET.

CASE HISTORY

Dr. Serafina Corsello, M.D., founder and director of the Stress Center in Huntington, New York, and New York City, relates the story of Sarah, a 67-year-old woman. Dr. Corsello said, "Sarah came to me complaining of feeling 'stressed out.' She reported extreme mood swings, with frequent exaggerated perceptions of threatening events. Sarah was a noninsulin-dependent diabetic, needing to rely on her diet for control. Like all diabetics, she loved sugar. As her poorly-regulated sugar levels see-sawed, creating floods of insulin and mood swings similar to floods of adrenalin, she experienced fatigue, sweats, dizziness, headaches, and disorientation. Because insulin is lipogenic (fat-producing), her cholesterol level was 320, and triglycerides, 225.

"I prescribed 800 micrograms of GTF chromium. Diabetics need at least 600 to 800 micrograms, especially if they are overweight. Sarah weighed 250 pounds.

"I instructed Sarah to eat five small meals daily, instead of three larger ones, with emphasis on fish and vegetables. The change in diet helped to eliminate her distended stomach and her cravings for sugar. Eating large meals triggers receptors which in turn trigger insulin production, creating up-and-down mood effects. In two weeks, Sarah lost weight, and began to feel human again. Today, Sarah's blood sugar metabolism, lipid profile, *and moods* are in total harmony."

THERE IT IS:
GTF CHROMIUM FOR THE RELIEF OF STRESS.

Comparison of Trivalent Chromium

Biological Properties	Simple Cr Compounds	GTF Chromium
Potentiation of insulin	+	+++
Effect on impaired glucose tolerance	+	++
Intestinal absorption	0.5%-3%	10%-25%
Access to physiological chromium pool	-	+
Placental transport	-	+
Toxicity	>	<

CHAPTER 6

HEART HEALTH

why you lose it, how you keep it

GLOSSARY

cardiovascular - relating to heart (cardio) and blood vessels (vascular); arteries in particular.

cholesterol - lipid continually manufactured and destroyed in the body.

> *HDL cholesterol* - fraction of blood containing fats and proteins; associated with reduced risk in heart disease.
>
> *LDL cholesterol* - fraction of blood containing fats and proteins; associated with increased risk in heart disease.

lipoproteins - molecules consisting of lipid joined to a protein.

triglycerides - principal type of fat stored by body as reserve fuel; one of risk factors for cardiovascular disease usually elevated when blood glucose is elevated.

CHROMIUM AS HEART HEALTH HELPER

One in a thousand care to take the trouble;
the others let the trouble take them.

HEART HEALTH: WHAT IT IS

THE KILLER DISEASE

A few years back, two of my brothers-in-law died, each at a young age—in the prime of their lives. Heart attacks.

Heart disease is still the number one killer. In fact, it accounts for a greater number of fatalities than all other diseases combined.

My interest in the subject goes beyond my work as a researcher and nutrition educator. I still feel the loss of my close relatives, and, just this last year, of two intimate friends.

WHAT ABOUT CORONARY BY-PASS?

Heart disease caused by atherosclerosis means that fat and cholesterol deposits have built up in your arteries, enough to place you at death's door. Not to worry, say the traditional physicians: the coronary by-pass procedure was developed to allow your circulation to by-pass the clogged up areas. You probably know at least one person who has had this surgery.

Although the operation has not entirely fulfilled its promise, it is still widely performed.

The very tests preceding the surgery are highly invasive, and the operation itself is major. Catheters inserted, tubes threaded from every orifice, electrodes attached, blood withdrawn, monitors recording every beat, drugs administered, vein(s) harvested from your own leg, complex heart-lung machines at the ready, rigging with stainless steel wires to help put Humpty Dumpty back together again. These measures are all part of this "common" application to restore your heart health. No one will tell you what you don't need to know, part of which is: *all of this technology is not always foolproof.*

Yet if you are male and between the ages of thirty-nine and fifty, the chances are horrifyingly good that a doctor will recommend that you undergo exactly this procedure sometime in the next twenty years. Women, although not as susceptible, are not exempt either. It is possible that the bypass operation, however invasive, may have extended the lives of my in-laws, even though it did not work for my two friends.

THE GREATEST ADVANCE IN MEDICINE HAS NOT BEEN IN THE DISCOVERY OF NEW DRUGS OR IN THE HIGH TECHNOLOGY OF THIS ERA, BUT IN *PREVENTION.*

Just how difficult is prevention? Can we practice a disease-preventing lifestyle without giving up the pleasures of late twentieth century rewards? I think we can.

SYNDROME X

At the Banting Lecture Series, an important annual symposium, an interesting constellation of events was presented to a large group of physicians. The cluster of occurrences described by the experts was called *Syndrome X*. It starts with *insulin resistance* and continues in this order: glucose intolerance, too much insulin, increased levels of triglycerides, increased levels of harmful very-low density lipoprotein (LDL), decreased levels of beneficial high-density lipoprotein cholesterol (HDL), and finally, *hypertension*.[1] The negative correlation between HDL and insulin suggests that low HDL, like high triglyceride levels, is a manifestation of insulin resistance.[2]

MAINSTREAM MEDICINE IS BEGINNING TO RELATE BLOOD SUGAR METABOLISM WITH HEART PROBLEMS!

What do we know about heart disease? Can this kind of knowledge and other current information help to prevent the number one killer? Researchers say *yes*. To understand what heart health is, we'll discuss what it isn't.

CHROMIUM AND HEART DISEASE

We know that chromium deficiencies have been implicated in most of the factors of cardiovascular risk. Levels of chromium in those with coronary artery disease are much lower than in healthy people.[3] If chromium deficiency is a primary risk factor for coronary heart disease, would chromium supplementation be of benefit?

Previous chapters discussed the correlation between the deficiency of this trace mineral and impaired sugar and fat metabolism. The relationship between chromium shortages and high levels of circulating insulin has been explained. The literature indicates that chromium may also help to prevent the buildup of plaque in arteries by lowering low-density lipoprotein cholesterol, and increasing high-density lipoprotein cholesterol. The key factor is chromium's remarkable ability to stimulate insulin action.

TOO MUCH INSULIN AND HEART DISEASE

Too much blood insulin, called *hyperinsulinemia*, appears to be a major component in heart disease. Those with elevated insulin usually have high LDLs, low HDLs, and high blood pressure.[4] Insulin stimulates your body's production of an enzyme that causes your liver to produce cholesterol. An oversupply of insulin in your blood could incite changes in the arterial walls that promote the formation of fatty plaques—your introduction to coronary heart disease.

High blood insulin may also explain why Type II diabetics, who produce plenty of insulin but don't utilize it properly, are two to four times more likely to develop heart disease than non-diabetics. (More on high blood insulin and diabetes in Chapter 7.)

Too much insulin favors salt and water retention, both of which also increase your risk for heart disease. In addition, high insulin levels can aggravate hypertension by intensifying the responsiveness of arteries to adrenaline.[5]

Unfortunately, unless patients exhibit symptoms of diabetes or hypoglycemia, most physicians do not test for elevated insulin. Yet the cumulative data linking insulin resistance with hypertension and risk factors for coronary artery disease are mounting.[6] Hyperinsulinemia is believed to result from insulin resistance—an inability to utilize insulin properly.

CHOLESTEROL LEVELS, CHROMIUM, AND HEART DISEASE

Studies indicate that LDL cholesterol promotes atherosclerosis, whereas HDL cholesterol exerts a protective effect.[7,8,9] This is in accord with observations of primitive societies, where cardiovascular disease is rare, and typical HDL/LDL ratios are high.[10,11]

Reasons for decreased chromium levels in western societies have already been discussed. More primitive groups have chromium levels two to three times higher than ours, and are relatively free of cardiovascular problems.[12] Based on these facts, can we assume that one of the reasons for heart disease is chromium deficiency? Although correlation does not prove causation, the evidence is overwhelming. But we don't have to second-guess. Scientific evidence proliferates.

VALIDATING CHROMIUM DEFICIENCY AND HEART DISEASE

Studies reveal the following information:

»Chromium deficiency increases serum cholesterol levels and the formation of aortic plaques. The feeding of chromium appears to prevent both the formation of such plaques and the rise of cholesterol—particularly the increase in cholesterol that takes place as you age. This information was reported in the *American Journal of Physiology*.[13]

»Chromium supplementation resulted in a 10 percent reduction of total cholesterol in those receiving chromium-rich brewer's yeast for two months. At the same time, beneficial HDL cholesterol increased by 14 percent, as described at the *Proceedings of the 5th International Symposium on Atherosclerosis* in Houston, Texas.[14]

»A study cited in *Diabetes* demonstrated significant decreases in cholesterol and insulin output in those fed brewer's yeast. A control group received chromium-deficient Torula yeast, to no avail.[15]

»Test animals given daily injections of chromium showed a significant regression of atherosclerotic plaques; control animals injected with water didn't exhibit any improvement. This was reported in the *American Journal of Clinical Nutrition.*[16]

»Autopsies establish that the aortas of people who die because of atherosclerosis usually lack chromium. This statistic is not true of people who die accidentally, as reported in the *Journal of Chronic Diseases.*[17]

»Low concentrations of chromium in hair and blood occur more frequently in those with cardiovascular disease. (Study cited in *Clinical Chemistry.*)[18]

»In response to chromium supplementation, HDL increases while circulating insulin tends to decrease. Researchers stated the following in the *American Journal of Clinical Nutrition:* "Chromium deficiency appears to be one factor in atherosclerosis."[19]

»The *American Journal of Clinical Nutrition* notes that a group of men taking 200 micrograms of chromium per day showed an 11 percent increase in HDL cholesterol. If insulin levels were too high at the outset of this study, chromium supplementation succeeded in lowering them.[20]

»Chromium supplementation of test animals fed diets of refined sugars, which are associatied with elevated cholesterol, has been reported to decrease these levels dramatically.[21,22] As cited in *Circulation*, an inverse correlation between HDL and plasma glucose has been noted in several epidemiological studies: lower glucose, higher HDL.[23]

Is there any doubt that chromium supplementation lowers total cholesterol and increases HDL? Is there any doubt about its use in the face of heart disease?

MORE ABOUT THE NIACIN CONNECTION

In 1983, the Journal of the American Medical Association published its findings on the accepted dietary and drug therapy for heart disease.[24] The report stated that high doses of the B vitamin niacin lower LDL and increase HDL. Studies confirmed the dramatic effects. Niacin can lower LDL cholesterol by as much as 30 percent and can increase HDL cholesterol up to 15 percent.

The use of niacin was popularized by Robert E. Kowalski's book, The 8-Week Cholesterol Cure. The problem is that megadoses of niacin are required to achieve the desired effect. Doses between 1500 and 3000 milligrams are suggested, which is 75 to 150 times that of the Recommended Dietary Allowances (RDAs). Niacin in such high amounts may result in serious side effects.[25]

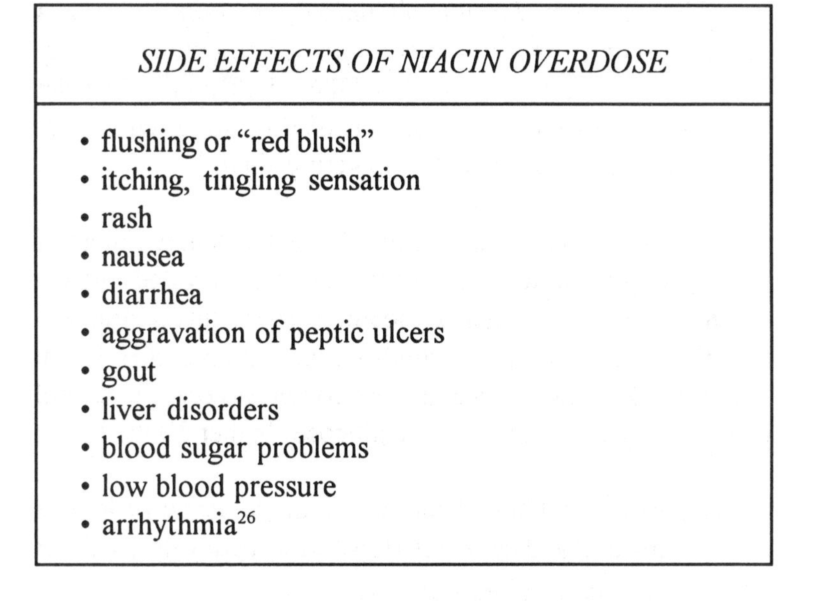

SIDE EFFECTS OF NIACIN OVERDOSE

- flushing or "red blush"
- itching, tingling sensation
- rash
- nausea
- diarrhea
- aggravation of peptic ulcers
- gout
- liver disorders
- blood sugar problems
- low blood pressure
- arrhythmia[26]

High doses (three grams or more daily) of timed-release niacin have been specifically indicted as being dangerously liver-toxic.[27] Some researchers believe that the mode of action that causes the problem is niacin's ability to release free fatty acids from your body's fat stores.

According to Mark Mitchell, Jr., M.D., associate professor of medicine at Johns Hopkins University School of Medicine, the way in which niacin lowers cholesterol is not completely clear. "It may be related to changes which control cholesterol synthesis, and we've seen elevations in liver enzymes in patients taking as little as two grams of [niacin] daily. But the majority of instances of liver toxicity has occurred in those taking more than three grams of timed-release niacin per day," states Dr. Mitchell.[28] It should be noted that niacinamide, a form of niacin that doesn't cause flushing, does not have a cholesterol-lowering effect.

CHROMIUM DIMINISHES
THE AMOUNT OF NIACIN
NECESSARY TO REDUCE CHOLESTEROL.

Dr. Martin Urberg, researcher at Michigan Wayne State University, discovered that when niacin and chromium are taken simultaneously, the amount of niacin required is significantly reduced.[29] Urberg demonstrated that a combination of 200 micrograms of chromium and only 100 milligrams of niacin results in as much as a 30 percent decrease in LDL cholesterol. He suggests that niacin and chromium work by the same mechanism. *Chromium and niacin lower insulin levels by providing the materials your body uses to manufacture its own GTF chromium.* Dr. Urberg discovered that when supplementation is discontinued, cholesterol levels rise. When supplementation is reinstituted, the level decreases. These findings are not surprising. Remember that Dr. Mertz identified the chromium-niacin complex as the primary component of GTF activity more than twenty years ago.[30] Taking additional niacin may not even be necessary when the chromium supplement has been preformed with niacin.

Dr. Richard Anderson of the United States Department of Agriculture stated that many people do not have the ability to convert inorganic chromium to the active GTF form.[31]

POPULAR CHOLESTEROL-LOWERING DRUGS

A word of caution for those using lovastatin as a cholesterol-lowering drug: its use raises a concern about liver health and the potential alteration of lymphoid cell function.[32] Ironically, some studies show that the cholesterol-lowering effects of lovastatin are too slight to be significant.[33]

EXERCISE AND HEART DISEASE

In 1984, it was established that death from coronary heart disease in those who regularly engage in moderate exercise was nearly 40 percent less than among nonexercisers.[34] A five-year follow-up of 3,000 fire fighters and police officers revealed that the incidence of heart disease doubled in a group with low fitness levels.[35] This is not news. But there is an obvious gap between the forward thrust of basic science and the shuffle with which the new knowledge is applied to human problems.

THE MINIMUM AMOUNT OF EXERCISE THAT IS HEART-PROTECTIVE DOES NOT INVOLVE TOO MUCH COMMITMENT: TWENTY MINUTES, THREE TIMES A WEEK.

Activity must be aerobic, or create breathlessness, but not pain or discomfort.[36] Check with your physician regarding the addition of GTF chromium to make your exercising habits easier and more beneficial. (Chapter 8 describes a simple, easy, and effective exercise program.)

HEART ATTACK RISK LIST

Risks for heart disease are listed, posted, reverberated, blasted, and stated yet again. You can probably recite some of these in your sleep: smoking, lack of exercise, alcohol, cholesterol levels, and obesity. Other risk factors are more "medical," and usually go unnoticed until you are confronted with a physician's personal warning.

Included in this list are:

»high insulin levels
»diabetes
»oral contraceptives
»arterial wall conditions
»blood platelet stability

We have already discussed the impact of chromium on exercise, obesity, cholesterol, and insulin. And no one needs another sermon on the dangers of smoking. Let's briefly examine two of the other hazards and see how chromium fits into the picture.

Arterial wall condition. Artery walls are very sensitive to insulin. Too much insulin causes the over-production of cholesterol and triglycerides, and thereby, plaque formation in artery linings—leading to atherosclerosis.[37] It is possible that chromium deficiency could cause these tissues to become insulin-resistant. This could be a reason for high levels of circulating insulin.[38,39]

Oral contraceptives. The risk of stroke is about nine times greater for women who use oral contraceptives compared with those who do not. The frequency of heart attack is also much greater.[40]

Impaired glucose tolerance, high levels of circulating insulin, and insulin resistance are also common problems among contraceptive pill users.[41] Since chromium supplements improve glucose tolerance and normalize insulin levels, chromium may be beneficial in alleviating the harmful effects of oral contraceptives. AS MANY AS 77 PERCENT OF WOMEN ON ORAL CONTRACEPTIVES SHOW SOME IMPAIRMENT OF GLUCOSE TOLERANCE.[42]

Tongue in cheek, I recently presented a talk to a large audience in Malaysia, called *How To Kill Your Spouse And Get Away With It.* Among the suggestions was the idea of offering your mate a cholesterol-raising snack: a salami sandwich on white bread with a cola drink, sweet pickles, pie-á-la-mode, followed by coffee laced with two or three teaspoons of sugar. Will this work if he or she is taking chromium? *Chromium supplementation used on test animals who were fed diets of refined sugar has been reported to significantly decrease cholesterol levels.*[43,44] (That doesn't mean a junk food diet won't cause other problems. This is *not* a recommendation to pig out!)

SUMMARY

Chromium supplementation could have beneficial effects on hypertension, arrhythmias, and other cardiovascular risk factors such as obesity and contraceptive-pill use.[45] The correlations are clear. If blood sugar metabolism and insulin are involved, chromium plays a role. Any attempt to reduce the threat of heart disease involves management that affects this metabolism. We find ourselves back at square one: disease starts at a cellular level. Whatever you do to improve your heart health will also improve other aspects of well-being. And the converse is true. What you do to improve energy, fitness, weight status, stress levels, and so on, will also have a positive impact on your heart health.

ONE IN A THOUSAND
CARE TO TAKE THE TROUBLE;
THE OTHERS LET THE TROUBLE TAKE THEM.

CASE STUDY

At her doctor's request, Maria had her blood chemistry checked at the APL Laboratories in Pahrump, Nevada. Her cholesterol reading was 260, and her triglyceride level was a whopping 863. Maria made no changes in diet or lifestyle, with one exception: She took chromium polynicotinate for two and a half months. Then she repeated the blood chemistry testing. She now had a cholesterol level of 217, and a triglyceride level of 154. Maria's HDL level increased from 31 to 43.

Recall that chromium potentiates the effect of niacin, and that niacin helps to regulate cholesterol levels. This proved to be a very effective metabolic pathway for lowering cholesterol.

It isn't easy to do what needs to be done to improve life quality. Because the leading cause of death among diabetics is cardiovascular disease, it isn't easy to separate discussions of chromium and diabetes from chromium and heart disease, either. Chromium-deficient animals have impaired glucose tolerance and atherosclerotic plaques in their aortas. The next chapter investigates blood sugar levels.

THERE IT IS:
GTF CHROMIUM FOR YOUR HEART.

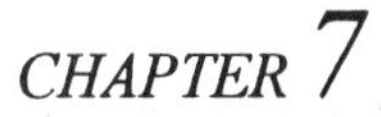

BLOOD SUGAR

what it is, how you control it

GLOSSARY

diabetes mellitus - disease in which blood glucose level exceeds normal range; characterized by inability to fully utilize glucose as energy source; commonly called "diabetes"; due to impaired insulin metabolism causing sugar to enter blood and urine.

> *Type I Diabetes* - insulin-dependent; usually caused by loss of function of most or all pancreatic B-cells.
>
> *Type II Diabetes* - noninsulin-dependent; the milder forms of diabetes; onset usually occurs after age 40; may be treated through weight control, dietary restrictions, and exercise.
>
> *Uncontrolled Type II Diabetes* - untreated; leads to kidney and eye disease and to twice the incidence of heart disease and stroke.

endocrine glands - glands containing tissues releasing hormones directly into bloodstream: thyroid, pancreas, adrenal, pituitary, others.

glucose tolerance - ability to lower blood glucose after its elevation by food ingestion; impaired in diabetes.

glycemic - the state of the presence of sugar in blood.

insulin - hormone secreted by B-cells of pancreas; required by most tissues to utilize glucose.

hyperglycemia - high blood glucose; elevation of blood glucose above normal range for given age and state of feeding.

hyperinsulinemia - excessive secretion of insulin by pancreas, resulting in hypoglycemia; insulin shock from overdosage of insulin.

hypoglycemia - low blood glucose; insulin reaction; insulin shock; may occur with or without gross clinical symptoms.

islets of Langerhans - cells in pancreas secreting insulin.

placebo - substance having no effect; administered for comparative control when testing active substance.

pancreas - large abdominal organ secreting insulin and other hormones into bloodstream.

CHROMIUM AS BLOOD SUGAR STABILIZER

There is no such thing as good medicine without attention to nutrition.

BLOOD SUGAR: WHAT IT IS

GTF CHROMIUM AND BLOOD GLUCOSE

A certain desert rodent, the sand rat, develops sugar diabetes when raised on laboratory food.

That's how the late Dr. Carl Pfeiffer, founder of the Brain Bio Center of Princeton, New Jersey, started his chapter on chromium in his best-selling book, *Mental and Elemental Nutrients: A Physician's Guide.* He went on to say:

When the sand rat is returned to the desert, its diabetic condition disappears. What is the key nutrient missing from rat food which the rat finds in its natural forage? Extensive laboratory analysis indicates that it is chromium. Chromium bound in an organic form in the glucose tolerance factor (GTF) potentiates the effect of insulin on glucose intake and so suppresses the latent diabetes of the sand rat. The salt-bush which is hoarded by the rat in its burrows contains enough GTF to prevent diabetes.[1]

NEWS RELEASE: SUGAR METABOLISM IMPROVED

Decade by decade, adult-onset diabetes (Type II) increases. It is estimated that almost 40 percent of the population over 60 is diabetic or borderline diabetic, and 80 percent over 65 are glucose intolerant to one degree or another.[2] The American Diabetes Association says *there are five million or more undiagnosed diabetics in the United States.*[3]

On April 3, 1990, the Federation of the American Societies for Experimental Biology, Office of Public Affairs, issued a news release. An excerpt of this news release follow.

Washington, DC: Chromium, a trace metal found at low levels in fruits, vegetables, bran and organ meats, improves sugar metabolism in about 85 percent of people who have a slight glucose intolerance and may be developing adult-onset diabetes, government scientists reported today at the 74th Annual Meeting of the Federation of American Societies for Experimental Biology.

In this study, [subjects] had mild glucose intolerance—their only sign of chromium deficiency—and were possibly developing adult-onset diabetes, said Richard A. Anderson, Ph.D., biochemist at the United States Department of Agriculture, Beltsville, Maryland.

Glucose intolerance is considered an early sign of adult-onset diabetes. It is usually not due to the inability of the pancreas to secrete insulin as in insulin-dependent, early-onset diabetes, but is caused by less effective insulin. The person's insulin shows less ability to control blood-glucose levels, causing the body to produce more insulin. Chromium increases the activity of the insulin, Anderson said.

More than 90 percent of the people in the United States have diets that provide less than the suggested safe and adequate intake of chromium, which is 50 to 200 micrograms per day, Anderson said. Furthermore, stress produced by high-sugar diets, trauma, or exercise, deplete the body of chromium. Chromium is toxic only at extremely high levels....

Chromium works as a nutrient, not as a drug; it affects only those subjects who are deficient in chromium, Anderson said. The chromium reverses glucose intolerance.

This essential trace metal, required at very low levels for the metabolism of sugar and fat, is not particularly high in any single food. People who do not consume sufficient dietary chromium, or who are slightly glucose intolerant, should take a balanced nutritional supplement that contains multi-vitamins and minerals, [continued Anderson]. Most Americans have low dietary intakes of several trace metals, especially chromium, copper and zinc.[4]

Additional information about this study appears on page 156 in the section on *Scientific Validation: Low Blood Sugar.*

GLUCOSE METABOLISM: REVIEW

If you remember your high school biology, or if you had reason to pay attention to glucose metabolism in later years (or to the preceding chapters of this book), you know that after you eat a meal, glucose is absorbed into your blood, causing insulin to be released by your pancreas. The insulin in turn causes rapid uptake, storage and use of glucose by almost all tissues of your body, but especially by your liver and muscles. Insulin helps with the storage of glucose in your liver as glycogen. And when you need to come up with some energy, liver glycogen is split back into glucose and released into your blood, where it is transported to various tissues in your body. Insulin affects fat and protein metabolism almost as much as it does carbohydrate metabolism.

THE ORGANIC GTF-CHROMIUM COMPLEX HAS BEEN IDENTIFIED AS THE BIOLOGICALLY ACTIVE FORM OF CHROMIUM.

Chromium itself has little effect on insulin. But in its biologically active form, chromium helps to bind insulin to cell-membrane receptor sites.[5] At these receptor sites, GTF-activated insulin works by transporting the blood sugar and vital amino acids into your cells for the metabolism of protein and carbohydrates. A lack of GTF chromium can inhibit this process, causing serious impairment of your physical development and performance.

Under normal conditions, when insulin is released into your blood, it doesn't last very long if it is not taken up by the targeted sites. In fact, if it doesn't bind to special places allocated for the purpose, it degrades in a matter of minutes. The problem is that "normal conditions" are rarely par for the course.

MORE ON INSULIN RESISTANCE

Although explained in previous chapters, the metabolism of chromium and blood sugar as it relates to insulin resistance bears repeating, especially in reference to diabetes. About 15 percent of the fifteen million people in this country with diabetes mellitus depend on insulin for life. Among the large percentage who have noninsulin-dependent diabetes, many are overweight and have insulin resistance. The insulin resistance may be caused by overweight or by the disease itself.

Insulin resistance is common not only in diabetes, but also

in those who are obese, have ovarian cysts, lupus or other autoimmune diseases characterized by antibodies to insulin receptors.[6] In other words, your body becomes immune to its own insulin, rejecting or neutralizing it.

ANTIBODIES CAN DESTROY INSULIN AT SUCH A FAST RATE THAT TEN TIMES THE AMOUNT OF INSULIN MAY BE REQUIRED BY SOME DIABETICS.

Insulin resistance may be caused by abnormally shaped or formed insulin molecules (the result of aging or free radical damage), sulphur deficiency, blockage of normal insulin function, and chromium deficiency.

Noninsulin-dependent diabetics may have plenty of insulin in their blood, but it is useless without GTF chromium to potentiate its activity. A gas station with tanks full of gasoline can not get a car going if the gas is not pumped into the tank.

INSULIN RESISTANCE TRANSLATES INTO INSULIN DEFICIENCY

No group of individuals is more susceptible to chromium deficiency than diabetics.[7,8] During the first twenty-four hours after a single oral dose of chromium, diabetics absorb two to four times more of this trace element than those with normal sugar metabolism.[9] When insulin is taken, 20 percent of the chromium mobilized from body stores is excreted. So administration of insulin may result in an increased excretion of chromium and a tendency to chromium deficiency, the last thing a diabetic needs.[10]

It's another vicious cycle:

»high blood sugar causes chromium loss
»which causes blood sugar to be high
»which causes chromium loss.

Because diabetics can't construct GTF from the component parts, they need to take chromium in an already-complexed GTF form.

> LESS INSULIN IS REQUIRED TO KEEP GLUCOSE CONTROLLED WHEN ADEQUATE GTF CHROMIUM IS PRESENT.

DISCOVERY OF INSULIN

The discovery of insulin more than 65 years ago revolutionized the treatment of diabetes. Despite the best efforts of the medical community, however, diabetics continue to have devastating complications. One of the most fundamental questions in diabetology is whether or not these side effects can be prevented or reversed by intensive insulin therapy.[11] According to recent studies, the replacement of insulin is an elusive goal despite important advances in our understanding of insulin's properties.

Studies by researchers at the University of Texas in Dallas conclude that physicians are not always able to normalize the elevated plasma glucose levels caused by insulin deficiency or insulin resistance. Their efforts often produce *hyperinsulinemia* (too much insulin).[12]

Insulin resistance can be the consequences of several factors:

»A decrease in the number of locations on cell membranes that accept insulin
»Chromium deficiency, preventing the insulin receptors from being able to accept insulin
»Defects in the cell that interfere with insulin's action.

Hypoglycemia is by far the most serious and common adverse *reaction* to the administration of insulin. With prolonged use of insulin, the natural hormonal checks and balances become ineffective.[13]

HYPOGLYCEMIA AND THE GLUCOSE TOLERANCE TEST

I will never forget my reactions during my glucose tolerance test—a six-hour trial to determine the effects of a potent dose of simple carbohydrate. The endocrinologist administering the examination told me that he was able to predict patients' blood sugar values as he inserted the needles. Experience taught him how to interpret the results from observation of blood vessel responses as he drew blood. He proved to be right in my case when he told me that I was going to break his records for low blood glucose readings. I exhibited severe hypoglycemia.

During the fifth hour of testing, I was so hungry and out of control that I wanted to eat the plants in the waiting-room aquarium. Another patient stopped me, pointing out that the plants were artificial. "I don't care," I said, "I must have something to eat. What about the fish?"

The oral glucose tolerance test has been criticized for subjecting people to an unreal situation. For me, the experience was not exaggerated. I had suffered similar reactions many times before. In fact, I had probably experienced the uncomfortable symptoms of low blood sugar for about ten years, never fully understanding why I felt so drowsy about an hour *after* eating (endogenous insulin dropped sugar levels lower than intended), or so antsy *before* eating—when my low blood sugar status signalled for glycogen breakdown, but my system was not computing.

BLOOD GLUCOSE: HOW YOU CONTROL IT

BREWER'S YEAST: CHROMIUM "SUPPLEMENT"

The history of GTF and its action on insulin goes back at least a century, although it was not exactly recognized as such. More than a hundred years ago, large amounts of brewer's yeast were fed to diabetics with great success, keeping the disease under control. The health benefits of brewer's yeast were perceived despite the lack of identity of any of its specific constituents. In 1929 two researchers noted the effect of yeast on the sugar-lowering action of insulin.[14] At that time, the advantages of brewer's yeast were attributed to its high nutrient content.

In the 1940s, women living in urban areas were discouraged from breastfeeding. My children and I were victims of this misguided philosophy. When I questioned my obstetrician about breastfeeding, his response was, "You are not a cow." The formula prescribed for my baby contained Carnation Milk, with a high sugar content. It is no surprise that my first child was dangerously ill by the time she was four months old. Having gained a limited knowledge of nutrition because of her illness, I began to add a tablespoon of brewer's yeast to every bottle fed to her. That was the end of any illness. My child thrived!

Looking back, it was a risky move on my part. Fortunately, she had a cast-iron stomach and was able to tolerate the yeast. I would not advocate this elixir in today's world for any child so young. Infants do not produce the enzymes necessary to digest anything other than mother's milk until they are at least eight or nine months old. (Offering foods before then creates food sensitivities that surface later on in life.)

Brewer's yeast was the best "natural" adaptogenic product I knew about at the time, and it worked. No doubt the chromium in the brewer's yeast was protective against the high percentage of sugar in the formula.

WEIGHT AND EXERCISE

It's more difficult for diabetics to lose weight because of the impasse in releasing fat from their cells. But diabetics must lose weight if they want to enhance their health and to be free of the disease. Getting rid of only five or ten pounds of fat curtails insulin requirements by a very significant amount. Muscle requires much less insulin.

EXERCISE BINDS GLUCOSE
WITHOUT THE NEED FOR INSULIN

According to Gary Price Todd, M.D., of Waynesville, North Carolina, every ounce of fat requires five times the amount of insulin than would be needed by muscle. So if you're only five pounds overweight, twenty-five times the amount of insulin is necessary compared with the quantity required for an extra pound of muscle. Weight loss helps to restore normal blood glucose.[15]

Diabetics who are not obese usually have idiosyncratic defects in insulin secretion.

Part of the metabolic adjustment that normally takes place during exercise is absent in insulin-dependent diabetics. A major problem is to reach *low but adequate* plasma insulin levels to maintain normal glycemic reactions during physical exercise. (Glycemia refers to the presence of sugar in your blood.)

In patients with low insulin levels and marked hyperglycemia, physical exercise may aggravate rather than ameliorate the diabetic state.[17]

In *hypoinsulinemic* patients, however, increased blood glucose levels may be seen in response to exercise.[18] Even those with normal glucose reactions suffer from decreased glucose concentrations with intense and prolonged exercise.[19]

CONTROL OF DIABETES: BREAKTHROUGH METHODS

Although chromium supplementation isn't as helpful for the insulin-dependent diabetic as it is for Type II diabetics, it often serves to modify the hypoglycemic effect. Dr. Todd uses chromium extensively in the treatment of diabetes. He has been able to get most of his Type II diabetics off their oral medications, and reduce the amount of insulin for the Type I patients. Dr. Todd explains that because chromium doesn't hang around very long in the diabetic—it just passes right through—diabetics require 600 micrograms with each meal, or at least 600 micrograms twice a day. (Please note: you must be under a physician's care if you take this quantity of chromium.)

Dr. Todd himself is an insulin-dependent diabetic. He was able to get his insulin down from 70 units a day to about 5 by taking 600 micrograms of chromium with each meal. Dr. Todd admits that if his diet was more exemplary, he could probably eliminate the need for insulin entirely. Although it is difficult to get Type I diabetics off insulin totally, Todd does have one patient with whom he was successful. This patient had previously required 20 units of insulin, and is now totally free of the need of any.

In the case of the diabetic, the high doses of chromium have to be continued forevermore (not without monitoring, of course.) For most other disorders, treatment with chromium involves high doses for therapy, and reduced amounts for maintenance.

CAVEAT FOR CLOSE RELATIVES OF DIABETICS

Impaired glucose metabolism is common in close blood relatives of patients with noninsulin dependent diabetes. They often exhibit a disturbance in glycogen formation.[20] So, relatives, keep a watchful eye!

DIABETIC RETINOPATHY (DISEASE OF THE RETINA)

In poorly controlled diabetes, *retinopathy*—a noninflammatory disease of the retina—takes the form of degeneration of the retinal blood vessels which show fluid leakage in early stages, and hemorrhages in late stages.

Poor control of blood glucose is thought to be an important factor in the development of diabetic retinopathy.

STUDIES SHOW A LINK BETWEEN DIABETIC CONTROL AND MICROVASCULAR COMPLICATIONS.[21]

DIABETES AND HEART DISEASE

Although HDLs are normal or high in well-controlled insulin-dependent diabetics, HDL levels are often low in noninsulin-dependent diabetes—a condition in which insulin resistance and defective insulin secretion are prominent features.[22]

Insulin functions can be enhanced by increasing insulin concentrations, and also by increasing biologically active forms of chromium. Keeping circulating insulin levels within normal range is especially beneficial because of the complications linked to diabetes. These include coronary heart disease associated with elevated insulin.[23]

Macrovascular disease is very common among diabetics. Current thinking associates insulin with the cause of this complication. Again—although there may not be a direct correlation between benefits for insulin-dependent diabetics and chromium supplementation, several indirect values have been suggested.[24]

HOW CHROMIUM HELPS THE DIABETIC

GTF chromium helps the diabetic in several ways. It is responsible for:

»a substantial decrease in insulin requirements for insulin-dependent diabetics

»a correction of abnormal glucose tolerance curves

»a normalization of elevated triglycerides in certain young adults
»significant reduction in cholesterol levels
»correction of impaired glucose tolerance in elderly subjects
»decreased insulin needs to maintain normal glucose tolerance

THE DIABETIC DIET

Views about food are often historic rather than scientific, and myths about sugar and energy appear to head the "science-by-press-release" list. According to researchers at the University of Vermont, we have been relying more on *tradition* than on *fact* in certain choices of diet treatment for hypoglycemia.[25] Orange juice, a commonly prescribed antidote for hypoglycemia, is not the most potent glycemic agent.

EQUAL AMOUNTS OF OTHER CARBOHYDRATE FOODS, SUCH AS WHOLE GRAINS (IN THE FORM OF CEREAL OR RICE), PRODUCE MORE SUSTAINED ELEVATIONS OF BLOOD SUGAR THAN ORANGE JUICE.[26]

Just as insulin is necessary to move glucose out of your blood and into your cells, it is also necessary for the same mobilization of triglycerides. One patient reported that eating fried foods raised his blood sugar more than eating a sweet dessert. Overloading on fat increases insulin requirements. Reducing fat (particularly fried foods), helps to reduce insulin needs.[27]

Asked if he recommends foods high in chromium, Dr. Todd stated that so-called high-chromium foods alone won't work—there isn't enough chromium in our food to be effective for therapy. He does caution the diabetic (and anyone else, for that matter) not to eat any sweet dessert at or after dinner, for reasons explained in Chapter 3. (Recall that growth hormone is produced at night; sugar interferes with its nocturnal release, thereby affecting your energy status, among other important functions dictated by this hormone.)

AN HOUR AND A HALF AFTER CONSUMPTION, A SINGLE EXPOSURE TO SUGAR INTAKE LEADS TO MARKED INCREASES IN CHROMIUM EXCRETION.

Losses persist as refined sugar continues to be eaten. (Again: once chromium is mobilized for use, it is excreted, rather than stored.) Needless to say, foods high in simple sugars replace nutritious foods which may have had other important vitamins and minerals, and perhaps at least some traces of chromium. Individuals with diabetes (and low blood sugar) respond differently to foods with equal carbohydrate and calorie content.

You already know that carbohydrates have different degrees of complexity, and that most simple sugars raise blood glucose rapidly. But some complex carbohydrates are converted to simple sugars merely by cooking.

THE LONGER A POTATO IS COOKED
THE MORE SIMPLE SUGARS IT CONTAINS
AND THE FASTER IT RAISES
YOUR BLOOD GLUCOSE.

Most packaged and restaurant soups contain considerable amounts of simple sugars or sucrose. Even soups prepared at home from fresh vegetables may contain high glucose levels if cooked for several hours.[28]

Blood glucose and insulin responses depend on particle size and cooking time as well as the type of cooking process.[29] Smaller particle sizes contribute to unwanted higher responses. (The rate of digestion is increased, and, with it, the subsequent increased glycemic responses.) This is why a bowl of whole grain cereal is far superior to pasta or even to whole grain bread or rolls. In the latter foods, the whole grain has been mushed, mashed, and mangled.

Consumption of legumes (peas, beans, and lentils) by diabetics results in improved glucose tolerance and blood sugar control.[30] Legumes are particularly useful in decreasing blood glucose responses compared with other high-fiber foods.[31]

BLOOD SUGAR, DIABETES AND PREGNANCY

Pregnancy is considered diabetogenic since abnormal glucose tolerance curves are observed in the majority of pregnant women during the last trimester of pregnancy. Normally, pregnant women maintain plasma glucose levels within a narrow range during the course of a day. But there is a marked increase in insulin after each major meal, and a lower fasting glucose level starting early in pregnancy. The low amounts are maintained until close to delivery, attributed to increased utilization of glucose by tissues. This level is significantly lower in malnourished women.

It is well known that latent diabetes may become unmasked during pregnancy. In addition to the needs of the fetus, high levels of circulating hormones are responsible for impairment in glucose tolerance. There is a correlation between low birthweight babies and growth retardation and poor glucose tolerance for the mother.[32] When glucose levels fall dangerously low, babies suffer mental retardation.[33] Disturbances of glucose metabolism in malnourished infants can sometimes be positively influenced by the addition of chromium to the formula.[34]

The high concentrations at birth suggest a selective mechanism for concentrating chromium from maternal sources by the developing embryo.[35] Dr. Carl Pfeiffer pointed out that many women in western countries are so deficient in chromium that the white blood cell chromium level may decrease by 50 percent with each pregnancy. This results first in complete alcohol intolerance, and later in glucose intolerance, leading to adult-onset diabetes.[36]

Severe hypoglycemia has been indicted as a potential cause for SIDS, sudden infant death syndrome. This information, reported in *Lancet*, is not surprising, but is the first scientific indication of such a correlation.[37]

Henry Schroeder, M.D., world authority on trace elements as they relate to living organisms, recommends 1.5 milligrams of chromium (1500 micrograms) daily during pregnancy.[38] Since this amount is several times higher than generally recommended by the National Research Council, pregnant women should consult their obstetricians about taking supplemental GTF chromium in this quantity.

WHEN SUGAR LEVELS ARE TOO LOW: HYPOGLYCEMIA

I wish I could explain with accuracy the precise causes, mechanisms and treatment for hypoglycemia, particularly because I am one of its many victims. Unfortunately, the etiology is not yet well established. Glucose intolerance is not specific for chromium, but if chromium deficiency prevails, glucose intolerance is almost always present.

I have been able to keep my symptoms to a minimum because I do not eat refined foods. I do not even consume natural foods with high amounts of simple sugars, such as fruit. I eat "intact" food, including raw salads laced with greens. I walk aerobically, and *do* or *don't do* whatever else is necessary for maintaining health. No lifestyle change, however, made as strong an impact on me as GTF chromium polynicotinate supplementation.

After several days on chromium, I was startled when I looked at the time as I sat working at my computer. "Something must be wrong with my clock," I thought. "Surely it can't be 1:30." My brain usually stops functioning long before noon: fatigue; hunger pangs; the sensation that I am a limp rag doll. These are the feelings that usually herald the hour for me around 11:00 AM. Somehow, this day was different. And it got better. The turnabout after three months can only be described as remarkable. Soon I was able to resume burning midnight oil, a practice I had long since discarded. In adaptogenic style, my improvement increased as time passed.

I checked personally with Dr. Michael Rosenbaum, Dr. Serafina Corsello, and Dr. Gary Todd Price, in addition to researching countless medical journal reports. My quest for information revealed similar experiences with many patients. The increase in insulin efficiency may be the precipitating factor in relieving symptoms of low blood sugar when chromium supplementation is administered. (Low blood sugar is often undetected because the tests administered for its presence are too brief.)

> IN ADAPTOGENIC FASHION, CHROMIUM HELPS TO MODIFY SUGAR LEVELS THAT ARE TOO HIGH OR TOO LOW.

SCIENTIFIC VALIDATION:
SUPPLEMENTING THE HYPOGLYCEMIC

Scientific validation of the chromium/low blood sugar paradigm surfaced with a fourteen-week study conducted by Dr. Richard Anderson and colleagues at the Beltsville Human Nutrition Research Center, Division of Endocrinology and Metabolism, Department of Medicine, at Georgetown University.

To determine if chromium is involved in low blood sugar, patients with symptoms of hypoglycemia were supplemented with 200 micrograms of chromium for three months in a double-blind crossover study: some of the patients received chromium, others a placebo that looked like the chromium supplement, and then the pills were reversed. Neither the subjects nor those administering the supplements knew who was getting what. The results proved that chromium supplementation alleviated the hypoglycemic symptoms.

The chromium supplementation:

»raised the minimum glucose levels
»improved insulin binding to red blood cells
»improved the number of insulin receptors
»reduced hypoglycemic symptoms

These findings demonstrated that impaired chromium nutrition and/or metabolism may be a factor in hypoglycemia.[39] The adaptogenic quality of chromium was fully demonstrated in these tests.

Results showed that chromium tends to:

»normalize blood sugar by decreasing it in those with elevated glucose values
»have no effect on blood sugar in those with near-optimal glucose tolerance
»increase blood sugar in those with low blood sugar

These consequences are most likely due to increased insulin efficiency.

For me, the most interesting aspect of the study was that the subjects *guessed with accuracy when they were getting the "real thing"* as opposed to placebo. Their improved feelings were the best clue! Patients who were normal or hyperglycemic could not differentiate between the chromium or placebo. But the low-blood-sugar people knew the difference. Impressive? You bet!

In another study, researchers gave 200 micrograms of chromium daily to 76 healthy humans and every one showed significant improvement: There was a 1,000 percent difference in chromium absorption efficiency.[40] Where was chromium when I took my glucose tolerance test years ago?

SCIENTIFIC VALIDATION: SUPPLEMENTING THE DIABETIC

The following information supports the use of GTF chromium supplementation for diabetics:

»The medical journal *Diabetes* reported that GTF chromium administration reduces elevated blood glucose to a normal level in both acutely and chronically diabetic test animals. Inorganic chromium is completely without effect.[41]

»Dr. Mertz demonstrated that small quantities of chromium are required for the optimal effect of insulin in every insulin-dependent system that has been investigated. Large concentrations of insulin are needed to achieve a normal response for chromium-deficient tissues.[42]

»Liver glycogen levels were significantly lower in test animals fed a low chromium diet than in those fed the same diet with supplemental chromium, as reported in the *Journal of Nutrition.* The test animals not given the chromium also had a decrease in glycogen formation in their livers and hearts following an intravenous insulin injection, as compared with the chromium-supplemented group.[43]

»Daily supplementation of 200 micrograms of chromium has been shown to normalize both hypoglycemia and hyperglycemia, as reported in the *Journal of the American Medical Association.*[44]

»Loss of chromium due to ionized iron may be one cause of adult onset diabetes. Widespread iron fortification in food, plus the addition of iron to multi-supplement formulas contribute to this problem. Chromium and iron are bound to the same blood protein, and excess iron displaces some of the chromium, which is then lost through the kidneys.[45]

CASE HISTORY

Dr. Rosenbaum reported that he sees a 10 to 20 percent drop in insulin requirements when his insulin-dependent diabetic patients supplement with 600 micrograms of chromium daily.

He related the story of Mark, whose blood sugar fasting level dropped 30 percent in a week. Dr. Rosenbaum cautions physicians and patients about the dramatic results: sometimes, insulin requirements decrease so rapidly that there could be danger of insulin overdose. He observes patients very carefully during the first week, and gives precise instructions for monitoring glucose levels until conditions stabilize.

SUMMARY

A few of the salient points relating to blood sugar discussed in this chapter are:

»Chromium helps to reverse glucose intolerance.
»Insulin can be enhanced by increasing biologically active forms of chromium.
»Noninsulin-dependent diabetics may be able to eliminate drug use with chromium supplementation.
»Insulin-dependent diabetics may be able to reduce insulin dosage.
»Exercise has a positive influence on blood sugar metabolism.

»The increase in insulin efficiency may be the precipitating factor in relieving symptoms of low blood sugar when chromium supplementation is administered.
»Insulin resistance is common not only in diabetes, but also in other disease states.

It must not be forgotten that *there is no such thing as good medicine without attention to nutrition.*

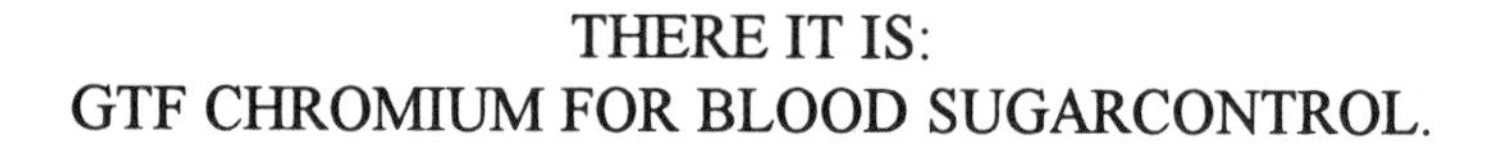
THERE IT IS:
GTF CHROMIUM FOR BLOOD SUGARCONTROL.

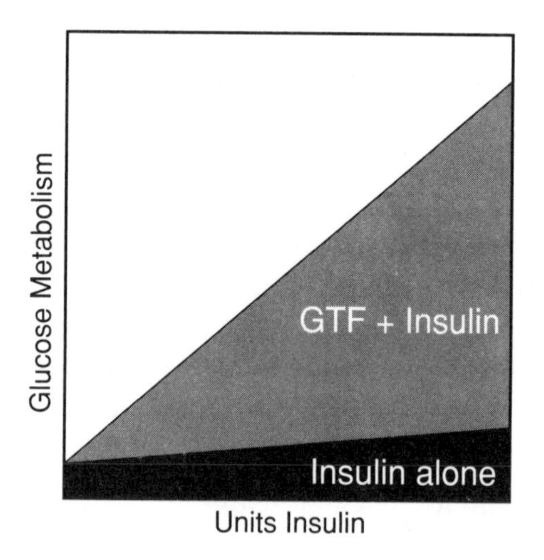

The next chapter puts it all together. It's the *how-to-do-it* chapter, strategy that can add joie de vivre for any one at any stage of life.

CHAPTER 8

STRATEGY

what to eat, how to supplement, how to exercise

GLOSSARY

diet - the food on your plate.

nutrition - what happens to the food on your plate.

optimal health - the best possible state of health.

polynicotinate - compound of niacin, as in *chromium polynicotinate.*

supplement - something added to supply a deficiency; reinforce or extend a whole.

STRATEGY

Food, exercise, supplements: these are among the few factors in your environment that you can control.

WHAT TO EAT

DOES YOUR DIET PROVIDE GOOD GLUCOSE METABOLISM?

Can you consume a diet that provides enough chromium as recommended by the National Academy of Sciences? Yes, if you are a Sumo wrestler! According to Dr. Anderson of the United States Department of Agriculture, more than 3,000 calories derived from a nutritious, well-balanced diet would have to be eaten to meet the ***minimum*** suggested intake, and more than 12,000 calories per day are needed to achieve the upper limit of 200 micrograms of chromium.[1] Anderson states that "there are no known foods eaten that are outstanding sources of dietary chromium." (Unless you dine with the sand rat on a salt-bush.)

The diet plan that makes the most sense is one that:

» includes foods that help to regulate blood sugar metabolism

»contains the least amount of the top allergenic foods

»does not include foods that have been extensively processed

FOOD FACTS AND SUGGESTIONS FOR IMPROVING GLUCOSE METABOLISM

In preparing the menu and recipe plan for improved glucose metabolism, the following information has been considered, and several suggestions noted:

»The lowest premature death rate is found in the Mediterranean area, which climatically favors a food supply of predominantly vegetable origin.[2]

»Ground rice (flour) produces a much greater glucose and insulin response than whole rice; puréed apples result in a greater response than whole apples; wheat in bread elicits a greater response than wheat in pasta; and pasta elicits a greater response than a bowl of whole grain cereal. Changing only one factor by cooking or processing alters your metabolic response. This factor is *food form*. The more intact the food is when it's on your plate, the more healthful your response.

The recommendation to augment fiber intake can best be carried out by an increased consumption of whole grain cereal products instead of foods made from low extraction flour—so you get the fiber and the healthful glucose management. More energy is lost than gained with the consumption of cereal fiber transformed into breads and rolls.[3]

»Sulphur-containing eggs may help glucose metabolism. The insulin molecule has four double bonds—eight atoms of sulphur. (Many anti-diabetic drugs are sulphur-containing.) Dr. Todd sees a connection here, and theorizes that this may be the reason he does not need additional insulin when consuming eggs, as described in Chapter 1. Eggs contain sulfur amino acids.

»Insulin is as necessary for the metabolism of *fat* as it is for *glucose*. The high percentage of fat in fried foods, plus the possibility of free radicals in these foods, requires more insulin for their metabolism.

»Slow digestion and absorption are factors that help protect susceptible people from developing diabetes.[4] Legumes are an excellent source of slowly digested carbohydrates.[5] (Legumes are peas, beans and lentils.)

»A diet emphasizing minimally-processed complex carbohydrate foods can be considered an aid to healthy glycemic responses. Fiber improves glucose tolerance.[6]

»Mung bean noodles (also known as *cellophane noodles*) elicit responses similar to those for raw products—they have lower glycemic and insulin reactions.[7]

»Change the potato into potato chips, and you convert 100 grams of fat-free, high-density complex carbohydrate into 500 calories of a mostly fat-type food. Oxidation of lipids could result in decreased utilization of glucose.[8]

Most of the nutritional elements of the potato are in the skin and eyes, from which roots and shoots grow. The rest of the potato is largely carbohydrate to supply nutrients until roots can take over and extract them from the soil.

»All whole raw foods, properly grown and consumed at peak, contain the micronutrients necessary for their metabolism in sufficient quantities.[9]

»Rather than gorging on a few chromium-rich foods, the best way to enhance your body's supply of chromium is to limit simple sugars, which cause excretion of large amounts of the mineral.[10]

»Special note to athletes: please consume liquids! You should be well-hydrated before a competition. Just don't drink much fluid *immediately* before an event.[11]

MENU AND RECIPE PLAN FOR IMPROVED GLUCOSE TOLERANCE

GENERAL RULES

The simplest and most healthful way to optimize glucose metabolism is to avoid elaborate recipes. Keep it simple; use *intact* foods. First, the negatives:

YOU SHOULD NOT EAT OR DRINK:

milk (whole), milk (skim or low fat), half-and-half, tea, coffee, de-caf, tap water, cheese and other milk products, fruit juice, yogurt as a meal, head or iceberg lettuce, salt butter, margarine, dried fruit, citrus fruit, ice cream, pretzels, canned soup, potato chips, wheat germ, bran, white bread, white rice, supermarket whole wheat bread, bottled oils, nuts that have been shelled (unless sprouted), cola, diet soda, cake, cookies, crackers, canned or frozen anything, sugar, salt, honey, processed flour.

What's left?

»YOU *CAN* EAT:
• eggs (fertile only; poached, boiled, or sunny-side-up are best)
• sweet butter (in very small amounts)
• these whole grains: millet, brown rice, buckwheat—with cinnamon, small amounts of fruit, and/or yogurt, but no milk
• Essene bread (made from sprouted grains)
• small amount of viable yogurt or acidophilus with each meal (2 tablespoons)
• cold-water fish (eat the skin too!)

»YOU *MUST* EAT:
vegetables—vegetables—vegetables—a lot! a lot! a lot! EVERY DAY—A LOT! Raw. Lightly steamed. Raw. As much as the appetite and digestion tolerate. You cannot overdose on vegetables. LEAFY GREENS: parsley, water cress, bib or romaine lettuce, arugula, spinach, kale, etc.

»YOU CAN ALSO EAT:
• fruit in moderation
• condiments—all kinds; onions and garlic are excellent

FRUIT FORMULA
1 fruit to 3 portions of vegetables (or 2 to 6). First, eat 3 portions of vegetables. Then you may have one fruit, preferably an apple or a banana. Ideal: 6 portions of vegetables daily, and two fruits.

»YOU SHOULD EAT:
- foods to reduce toxic levels
  (especially for city folk):
- 1 cup peas or beans daily
  (string beans, green peas, lentils, etc.)
- ½ cup alfalfa sprouts daily
- lots of raw vegetables

BREAK A CAPSULE OF GTF CHROMIUM INTO THE WATER IN WHICH YOU SOAK YOUR SPROUTING SEEDS.

»BEVERAGES

If herb teas are unpalatable, add unprocessed apple juice until taste buds are reeducated. Diminish the amount of juice until it is no longer needed. Add cinnamon or a cinnamon stick to herb tea. Drink lots of water (pure, of course).

»ESPECIALLY GOOD FOODS

Bananas (if no low blood sugar), Lima beans, sweet potatoes, avocados, vegetable broths (homemade), millet, brewer's yeast, liver and other organ meats, tempeh and tofu, homemade vegetable blends, deep sea fish, sunflower seeds (purchased in the shell, unsalted, unroasted).

Some people respond to diet changes immediately. Others require several months before feeling better. There are those who even feel worse before improving. But there is a pot of gold at the end of this rainbow.

SPECIFIC MENUS WHICH MAY BE HELPFUL

In addition to healthful glucose metabolism, elimination of allergenic foods, and foods with minimal processing, the following factors should also be considered in the menu plan:

- *variety*
- *quality protein* (not necessarily quantity)
- *quality fiber*
- *convenience*

Most people have neither the time nor inclination to follow recipe plans. And that's okay. These menus and recipes are for those who have lots of time, lots of money to hire a chef, or are simply looking for a few new ideas. (Recipes follow Day 7.)

»Day 1
Breakfast: 2 poached eggs; rice cakes with butter; apple
Lunch: lentil soup;[a] large salad[b]
Dinner: liver slivers;[c] lots of lightly steamed vegetables[d]

»Day 2
Breakfast soy pancakes;[e] small banana
Lunch: tarator soup;[f] large salad[b]
Dinner: steamed chicken (organic);[g] lots of lightly steamed vegetables[d]

»Day 3
Breakfast: millet with cinnamon and banana slices[h]
Lunch: chicken salad;[i] Essene bread
Dinner: broiled fish;[j] lots of lightly steamed vegetables[d]

»Day 4
Breakfast: eggs, sunnyside up; grated carrot[k]
Lunch: string bean mousse;[l] large salad[b]
Dinner: oriental brown rice;[m] lots of lightly steamed vegetables[d]

»Day 5
Breakfast: buckwheat pancakes with apples[n]
Lunch: tofu omelet;[o] salad[2]
Dinners: salmon trout;[p] lots of lightly steamed vegetables[d]

»Day 6
Breakfast: avocado omelet[q]
Lunch: fish salad;[r] large salad[b]
Dinner: the "Soup" [s]

»Day 7
Breakfast: granola (wheat- and milk-free)[t]
Lunch: egg foo yung with tofu;[u]
Dinner: curried rice;[v] lots of lightly steamed vegetables[d]

EVERYDAY STAPLES
• SPROUTED SUNFLOWER SEEDS (PURCHASED UNHULLED, UNSALTED) • RAW VEGETABLES FOR NIBBLING (CARROTS, CELERY, GREENS) • SMALL QUANTITY OF YOGURT

»Everyday options: herb tea; sunflower lettuce or other nutrient-dense greens

RECIPES

(a) **Lentil Soup**

¼ cup olive oil
2 medium onions, diced
2 stalks celery, diced
6 cups water
1 cup lentils, rinsed
8 oz tomato sauce (preferably homemade)
2 cloves garlic, minced
fresh ground pepper to taste

Pour olive oil into large skillet; sauté onions and celery until translucent. Add lentils to 6 cups water. Add tomato sauce, garlic, pepper, sautéd onions, and celery. Stir. Bring to boil. Cover. Simmer on low 1¼ hours. Can be prepared ahead—even the day before. Add slices of chicken or turkey "franks" to soup if desired.

(b) **Salad**

A salad is an incongruous, heterogeneous, or haphazard mixture. Based on this true definition of a salad, no two salads should be identical. Salads for improving glucose metabolism contain at least 6 ingredients. Mix and match:

red and/or green pepper, onion, green peas,
leafy green lettuce, parsley, water cress, grated carrot,
grated or diced zucchini, cabbage, garlic, sunflower seeds,
avocado, cucumbers, broccoli, asparagus, sesame seeds,
endive, arugula and sprouts.

No other foods are as nutrient-dense as home-grown sprouts. Add alfalfa, radish, wheatberry, red clover, mung, chick-pea, rye, sunflower, lentil, azuki.

(c) **Liver Slivers**

½ lb liver
½ onion, sliced thin
butter or oil
1 apple, sliced thin

Slice liver into thin, spaghetti-sized strands. Simmer onions in butter or oil; add liver and apple slices. Stir-fry quickly, moving pieces about while cooking. Do not overcook. This is a fast process. (Serves 1 or 2)

(d) **Steamed Vegetables**

If you don't have a large steamer pot, buy an inexpensive steamer basket that makes a steamer of any pot you own with a cover. Steam only until veggies reach prime color—still crisp. Slice those veggies which cook quickly into thick pieces (zucchini, etc.); cut smaller chunks of slower-cooking varieties (squash, sweet potato, etc.). Steam: broccoli, squash, cabbage, zucchini, string beans, onion, Brussels sprouts, sweet potato, peppers, green peas.

(e) **Soy Pancakes**

3 eggs
4 tablespoons soy flour
1 cup hot water
oil for pan
lemon juice and mashed fruit for topping

Blend eggs and soy flour until smooth and thick. Put in bowl and stir in enough hot water to make thin batter. Transfer to pitcher. Brush hot pan with oil and pour in enough batter to make thin pancake. Brown on both sides; fold in two. Set cooked pancake aside on hot plate until cool. Serve with lemon juice and mashed sweet fruit mixed together. (Serves 2)

(f) **Taratori Soup**

4 oz shelled walnuts
5 peeled garlic cloves
5 teaspoons olive oil
5 cups plain yogurt
½ cup cold water
1 medium-sized cucumber, peeled and diced
fresh parsley or dill

Mix walnuts and garlic. Add olive oil, a few drops at a time, stirring constantly, until smooth. In bowl, beat yogurt until smooth. Blend in walnut and garlic mixture and ½ cup cold water. Add cucumber. Chill in fridge. Serve cold, sprinkled with finely chopped parsley or dill. This is the best cold soup you've ever eaten. (Serves 6)

(g) **Steamed Chicken**

1 small organic chicken
1 teaspoon oregano
2 cloves garlic, minced
½ teaspoon paprika.

Place chicken in steamer basket over an inch or two of water. Bring water to boil. Steam on low heat for 30 minutes, covered. Remove chicken, cut into eighths. Dust with oregano and sprinkle with garlic and paprika. Broil until golden brown. (Serves 3 or 4)

(h) **Easy Millet**

1 cup water
½ cup millet
cinnamon
banana, sliced.

Boil water; add millet. Lower heat; cook, covered, 15 to 20 minutes, or until all water is absorbed. Add dash of cinnamon and sliced banana. (Serves 1 or 2)

(i) **Chicken Salad**

Last night's leftover chicken; 1 stalk celery; seasonings to taste; homemade mayonnaise. Dice chicken; add celery and seasonings and mayonnaise to taste.

(j) **Broiled Fish**

1 green pepper
1 small onion
1 clove garlic
½ teaspoon minced ginger
butter for pan
fresh fish from deep ocean
½ cup sesame seeds
juice of ½ lemon
parsley for trim.

Simmer pepper, onion, garlic, and ginger in butter or oil. Place fish on top, and simmer for about 10 minutes. Sprinkle sesame seeds on top, and place under broiler until done. Add lemon juice. Embellish with crushed parsley. (Serves 2)

(k) **Grated Carrot**

2 small or 1 big carrot, grated
½ onion
sprouted sunflower seeds

Combine all. (Serves 2)

(l) **String Bean Mousse**

2 cups lightly steamed string beans
2 hard cooked eggs
2 tablespoons homemade mayonnaise
garlic
seasonings to taste

Toss all ingredients into food processor (or blender) and whip until light and frothy. (Using an eggbeater is okay too.) (Serves 2 to 4)

(m) **Oriental Brown Rice**

1 tablespoon sesame oil
1 cup brown rice
2½ cups water
1 cup mushrooms
2 cups bean sprouts
1 cup green peas
1 cup chopped scallions
1 cup diced water chestnuts
1 cup chopped celery
1 cup chopped green or red peppers
4 cloves mashed garlic
3 additional tablespoons sesame oil
1 teaspoon tamari
2 eggs.

Place 1 tablespoon oil in skillet and heat. Add rice slowly, with heat still on, stirring continuously until each grain is coated with oil. This only takes a few minutes, but prevents grains from sticking. Pour water into another pot. Bring to boil. Add oil-coated rice slowly and cover pot. Reduce heat to lowest possible setting. Cook 30 minutes. (No peeking; don't let the steam out.) Stir-fry mushrooms quickly; set aside.

Add remainder of ingredients, except eggs and tamari. Stir-fry quickly. Add tamari. Add rice and stir all. Lightly scramble 2 eggs; toss into mix. Optional: add 1 or 2 cups diced chicken or turkey (only if organic). (Serves 4)

(n) **Buckwheat Pancakes**

2 eggs
2 ½ cups buttermilk
2 tablespoons butter
2 cups buckwheat flour
1½ teaspoons baking powder (aluminum-free variety) whole milk yogurt.

Combine eggs and buttermilk. Add butter, beat mix thoroughly. In separate container, stir together flour and baking powder, pressing out any lumps. Add liquid ingredients, stirring only until blended. Add water if too thick, more flour if too thin. Drop batter on slightly greased hot griddle. Cook until just a bit dry on top (bubbles will form); turn and cook on other side. Serve hot. Serve with yogurt. (Serves 4 to 6)

(o) **Tofu Omelet**

Butter for pan
1 green pepper, diced
½ cake tofu
½ cup mushrooms, diced
1 small onion, diced
5 eggs, beaten
alfalfa sprouts

Melt butter in pan. Simmer pepper, tofu, mushrooms and onions in butter. Add beaten eggs. Stir while cooking until eggs are done. Serve with alfalfa sprouts. (Serves 2 or 3)

(p) **Salmon Trout**
This fish is so good as is, all it requires is broiling with a little bit of butter and pressed fresh garlic.

(q) **Avocado Omelet**

butter for pan
2 eggs, beaten
¼ avocado

Heat pan with butter; pour in beaten eggs. Let eggs cook pancake style. Add diced avocado to one-half of pancake egg, folding over second half. Allow to heat through. (Serves 1)

(r) **Fish Salad**

last night's left-over fish
seasonings

Mix with seasonings as desired.

(s) **The Soup**

2 quarts water
½ cup rice (or barley or millet)
½ cup each: diced onion, green pepper,
celery, carrot, sweet potato, zucchini squash, mushrooms
dash pepper
clove crushed garlic
oregano, thyme, and basil, dried
1 tablespoon tamari

Bring water to boil. Add rice (or other grain). Reduce heat and cover. Cook over low heat for ½ hour. Add vegetables, seasonings and tamari. Barely simmer for 1 to 2 hours, or until ready to eat.

(t) **Granola (Wheat- and Milk-Free)**

rice flakes
toasted soy-nuts
pecans
rice flouroil
water
vanilla

Mix all in quantities according to taste.

(u) **Egg Foo Yung with Tofu**

1 cup alfalfa sprouts (or mixture of sprouts)
3 eggs, lightly beaten
6 ounces tofu, cut into small squares
½ green pepper, thinly sliced
¼ cup minced onion
1 teaspoon tamari
4 teaspoons oil
pepper.

Combine first six ingredients, mixing well. Heat 2 teaspoons oil in heavy skillet. Pour in one half of egg/tofu mixture to form thin omelet. Cook for 2½ minutes on each side until nicely browned. Repeat until all ingredients have been used. Top with pepper. (Serves 2 to 4)

(v) **Curried Rice**

2 tablespoons butter
1 medium onion, chopped
1 apple, cored and chopped
¼ cup raisins (soaked)
2 cups cooked brown rice
curry powder to taste
2 tablespoons chopped peanuts

Heat butter in saucepan. Sauté onion, apple, and raisins until tender. Add rice and mix. Stir in curry powder. Garnish with peanuts.

Variations: Use millet instead of rice; almonds or coconut instead of peanuts. (Serves 4 to 6)

FOR THOSE WHO WORK: SOME OF THESE LUNCHES CAN BE PREPARED THE NIGHT BEFORE.

If you would like additional health-oriented recipes, send a self-addressed stamped envelope to:

NUTRITION ENCOUNTER
BOX 2736
NOVATO, CA 94948

If we do not put the effort into health, we often have to put it into sickness. It's not easy to make changes, but, I hope you will agree that it's worth the effort.

And then there's the story of the man who never ate one crumb of food other than *natural*. He lived an exemplary lifestyle; he didn't even cheat on his birthday. When he died and went to heaven, he was served celery and carrot sticks, but he noticed that *down there*—in that *other* place, everyone was feasting on the most delectable gourmet foods. He complained to St. Peter.

"How come I've been given such meager pickings—especially after my most exalted food selections all through the years?" he asked.

St. Peter answered, "It doesn't pay to cook for two."

SUPPLEMENT STRATEGY: GENERAL

Although the focal point of this book has been chromium, supplementation with a range of nutrients can help most people improve immune status. I have always been a proponent of food-type supplements, such as algae or other green foods (chlorella, spirulina, barley green, etc.), acidophilus, garlic, essential fatty acids, brewer's yeast, bee pollen, food-grown nutrients, certain whole herb extractions, and so on. A general multi supplement, plus additional vitamin C with bioflavonoids, and perhaps specific nutrients for particular problems should be considered and discussed with your physician.

Supplements should always be introduced *one* at a time. It is easier to adjust to new supplements if they are added in small doses. Some "new" supplements have been around for a million years of time, but their availability in supplemental form is based on the high technology of this century.

Dr. Rosenbaum is widely recognized as a pioneer in the field of nutritional medicine. He has developed nutrient-supplement plans for particular needs. One general regime consists of vitamin A, 10,000 IU; carotene, 25,000 IU; thiamine, 50 mg; riboflavin, 50 mg; niacin, 50 mg; pyridoxine, 50 mg; pantothenic acid, 100 mg; folate, 400 mcg; $B_{12,}$ 100 mcg; biotin, 400 mcg; choline, 500 mg; inositol, 100-250 mg; vitamin C, 1,000-5,000 mg; bioflavonoids, 500 mg; vitamin E, 200-600 IU. He adds calcium, 500 mg; chromium polynicotinate, 200 mcg; magnesium, 250 mg; manganese, 10 mg; selenium, 100 mcg; and zinc, 30-50 mg. This is a program outlined in his best-selling book, *Super Supplements*.

Taking supplements should be considered as a secondary measure for good health. *The food you eat is primary.*

HOW TO SUPPLEMENT WITH CHROMIUM

A PROPHESY FOR HEALTH

It has been more than two decades since Dr. Mertz told us that the impairment of glucose tolerance could be prevented by the addition of chromium supplements to the diet, and reversed by a single oral dose of 20 to 50 micrograms of chromium.[12]

Fifteen years ago, Dr. Carl Pfeiffer stated:

We know that certain vegetables will form GTF when the soil is supplemented with the chromium ion. Perhaps further supplementation with niacin and chromium might allow more of the GTF to be formed. At last, the riddle is almost solved, and we look forward to the time when pure GTF will be available for use in hypoglycemic patients and diabetics.[13]

Too bad Dr. Pfeiffer isn't around to see his prophesy come true. Niacin-bound GTF chromium is widely available today. Dr. Pfeiffer knew that this kind of supplementation would serve as a potent nutritional strategy for increasing insulin output and enhancing its effects.

Since Dr. Pfeiffer's hopes, well-controlled studies involving human subjects have demonstrated beneficial effects of supplemental chromium on fasting glucose, glucose tolerance, blood lipids, insulin binding, and hypoglycemic blood glucose values and symptoms. Because chromium is a nutrient and not a therapeutic agent, it only benefits those people whose signs and symptoms are due to marginal or overt chromium deficiency—the adaptogenic effect. Almost everyone in the United States, however, shows at least some sign of chromium deficiency. It was mentioned earlier that tissue levels of chromium are lower in the United States than in other countries.[14,15]

While excessive levels of chromium are usually limited to industrial settings, lack of sufficient dietary chromium intake is widespread in the general population and can lead to serious health problems.[16] It's nice to know, too, that most people who use chromium supplementation report beneficial results.

THE REASON FOR CHROMIUM POLYNICOTINATE

Niacin, part of the B-complex (B_3) assists in the breakdown and utilization of fats, proteins and carbohydrates. In its role as coenzyme, niacin helps the oxidation of sugars and is essential to proper brain metabolism. By potentiating insulin, it also helps to regulate blood sugar levels.

Recall that niacin, the common name for nicotinic acid, has been identified by Dr. Mertz as the compound associated with GTF chromium's biological activity. Apparently, niacin is crucial for the formation of the proper molecular structure of GTF that facilitates insulin binding to cell membrane receptor sites. In other words, niacin-bound chromium or *chromium polynicotinate*, provides the correct key to unlocking insulin's powerful effects in your body.

Niacin can be bound to chromium in numerous ways, some more biologically active than others. The precise manner in which chromium and niacin are bound together is critical for its biological activity.

Following Dr. Mertz's lead, researchers at Massey University in New Zealand found that one form of chromium polynicotinate was eighteen times more active than other forms of niacin-bound chromium tested. The researchers determined that the molecular arrangement must resemble the part of the GTF structure that is recognized by the cell receptors or enzymes involved in the expression of the biological effect. In other words, the square peg must fit the square hole, and it's the GTF-chromium that has the right structure.[17]

As a result of Dr. Mertz's research, and that of other leading scientists, we now have considerable insight into the mechanisms of the glucose tolerance factor. This research has paved the way for the development of a better chromium supplement (chromium polynicotinate). Although the active substance in brewer's yeast was found to be the chromium-nicotinic acid complex, the precise structure remains to be determined.[18]

HOW MUCH CHROMIUM SHOULD YOU TAKE?

Here's the recommendation of the tenth edition of the RDA, released by the Food and Nutrition Board of the National Research Council, National Academy of Sciences:

Children	1 to 3:	20 to 80 micrograms
	4 to 6:	30 to 120 micrograms
	7 to 10:	50 to 100 micrograms
	11+	50 to 200 micrograms
Adults		50 to 200 micrograms

Note: Zinc and iron administered orally with chromium decreases chromium absorption.

CHROMIUM SUPPLEMENTATION: WHICH FORM?

When making your choice, consider these facts:

»Some people appear to lose their ability to convert inorganic chromium to a biologically active form.[19,20] Chromium deficiency can be combatted by increased intake of chromium, particularly of biologically active GTF, This points to the fact that the *kind* of chromium supplement taken is of vital importance.

»Much smaller amounts of GTF chromium are required to restore normal glucose tolerance than mixtures of brewer's yeast with inorganic chromium.[21]

»Hardly any uncomplexed chromium compounds can be found in natural sources, not even in water.[22] Dr. Mertz contends that natural complexes in the diet are absorbed better than simple chromium salts.[23] If you use a simple chromium salt, that is, chromium chloride, your body must change this to a form that is biologically available. Those who have the greatest need may have the most difficulty with the conversion process. Only one-half to one percent of inorganic chromium is absorbed.[24,25]

»Studies which demonstrate a lack of effect on glucose metabolism after chromium supplementation have almost always been conducted with inorganic chromium.[26]

»A small difference in the structure of the chromium complex makes a big difference in its biological activity and GTF effectiveness. The arrangement must resemble the part of the GTF structure which is recognized by the cell receptors involved.[27]

»There are limited studies demonstrating the positive results of chromium picolinate on muscle mass. Because of the paucity of information and a degree of skepticism, Dr. Anderson expects the United States Department of Agriculture to conduct its own studies.[28]

»Chromium polynicotinate had been tested extensively in animals and on humans for five years before being marketed to consumers. After that, it had been available strictly through doctors until its safety and efficacy were well-established.

»Chromium in its hexavalent form is toxic. Vitamin C helps to convert hexavalent chromium to a trivalent chromium.[29] This is some protection against toxic chromium from environmental pollution. But your body must be able to make that conversion. Another source of hexavalent chromium comes from the cooking of acid foods in stainless steel pots. Tomatoes and citrus fruit will pick up hexavalent chromium from stainless steel cookware.[30,31]

SUPPLEMENTING THE ELDERLY

Four out of ten elderly people normalized their glucose tolerance levels after treatment with 150 micrograms of chromium daily for four months.[32] Similar improvement, by the way, has been noted in middle-aged and younger Americans treated with oral chromium for periods of several months.[33,34] Since the elderly have difficulty absorbing nutrients, this is not a bad score. Perhaps the results would have been even better if the dosage had been increased.

SUMMARY

Given our sedentary lifestyles and the defects in our foodways system, a most important ingredient for increased stamina is that of supplementation with high energy-yielding, food-type boosters. Whether you want to stop feeling drowsy during the six o'clock news (or even at mid-day), desire to stay up past midnight to watch the late-late show, or strive to increase your next marathon score, supplementation may be able to increase your energy potential—regardless of how that energy force is to be expended.

HOW TO EXERCISE

WALKING WORKS WONDERS

This section is only for those of you who do not exercise. That probably means most of you. Only a minority of adults in our affluent society engages in appropriate regular physical activity.

Did you know that you get the same benefit out of thirty minutes of brisk walking as you get from twenty minutes of running? In fact, long periods of vigorous walking do more to reduce fat than brief sessions of jogging.[35]

Aerobic walking is the best possible exercise. Aerobic exercises are those that make your heart accelerate for a sustained period of time, causing a need for more air (oxygen). An aerobic exercise is go-go-go and not stop-and-go. It is important to keep up the exercise for a period of time—at least twenty minutes. If optimal benefit is the goal, you should exercise at least three or four times a week.

Treat yourself to a comfortable pair of shoes. Try the following plan in an effort to motivate yourself to exercise regularly:

Leave your house and walk five minutes. Turn around after five minutes and head back. Walk as fast as you can with comfort. You should not be walking so fast that you cannot carry on a conversation, but you should also feel slightly stressed. Do this for one week. Notice how far you've gone after five minutes. In a week, chances are you will have covered more territory than you did on the first day.

The second week, walk away seven minutes, then back. Continue to increase the time week by week, *slowly* working up to a minimum of twenty minutes daily.

By the time you reach your objective of twenty minutes (ten minutes out and ten back), you will probably want to walk for a longer period of time. Aerobic walking is addictive. You will be hooked. The important thing to remember is that the distance you go is far more important than the speed at which you travel.

When you are a seasoned walker, try experimenting with a few different types of motion:

(1) Pretend you are the Tin Man in *The Wizard of Oz*. You will walk with muscles more tense, and this will slow you down.

(2) Now see yourself as a rag doll, with your whole body loose, arms swinging freely, and taking larger strides. This Raggedy Ann or Andy mode is far better.

Walking uses muscles all over your body. Many muscle systems come into play when you walk.

AEROBIC WALKING:
• Delivers more oxygen to your muscles • Allows your lungs to get rid of more carbon dioxide • Increases tiny blood vessels throughout your body cells • Makes those same blood vessels more flexible • Increases bowel-function efficiency • Encourages better sleeping habits • Decreases fatigue • Lowers your blood pressure • Strengthens your heart • Lowers your triglyceride levels • Stimulates your lymph system • *Improves your glucose tolerance for better sugar metabolism*

Regular physical exercise may also be considered beneficial in the sense that it increases the quality of life.[36]

A walking program bolsters your ability to deliver nutrients throughout your body. It guarantees that both your body and eyes will be exposed to daylight. This causes an increased output of various glandular secretions.

Fitness can be achieved with continuous vigorous walking for regular periods of time each day, no matter what age you are or what level of activity or inactivity you participated in before starting.

The best way to assure compliance and dedication to a walking regimen is to meet a friend on the corner—a walking companion. You may skip your walk one day and disappoint yourself, but you won't disappoint a buddy.

EXERCISE FOR THOSE "OVER THE HILL"

You lose physiologic function of your organs at a rate of about 5 percent per decade after your thirtieth birthday. This is a natural consequence of aging. *These losses are similar to losses that occur additionally in those people who are inactive.* Even if you have never engaged in any physical activity, you can reverse some of the losses.[37] Physically trained individuals appear to have postponed, at least partially, the physical ravages of age.

The rate of adaptation to exercise slows as a person becomes older, and the recovery period following effort may be prolonged. The advice is to increase time, but not intensity, and allow for longer cool-down periods.

SUMMARY

Changing people's behavior is not easy. Such change tends to be short-lived and usually affect only those who are already health conscious and willing to respond to advice. To achieve greater benefits, new behavioral strategies are needed. I have not yet been able to determine precisely what those strategies are. But I do know that education is the beginning of change. (If I got my sister to walk, *anyone* is a candidate.) It is my hope that you learned enough to inspire you to make a few changes.

Food, exercise, supplements: these are among the few factors in your environment that you *can* control.

THERE IT IS:
GTF CHROMIUM FOR YOUR
GOOD-HEALTH STRATEGY

And so we learned that chromium may help if you:

»cannot lose weight
»want to have more energy
»participate in any form of athletics or aerobics
»are under stress
»overreact to ordinary circumstances
»have any problems with blood sugar metabolism (either too much or too little)
»sustain elevated cholesterol levels
»suffer from heart disease
»just want to insure your good health

You may want to discuss chromium supplementation with your physician. Or, since this is an age of self-help, you may want to consider the safe, minimum dosage of *chromium polynicotinate*, which is 200 micrograms daily.

REFERENCES: CHAPTER 1

[1] L Friberg and T Kjellstrom, "Cadmium," in *Disorders of Mineral Metabolism*, vol 1, eds F Bronner and JW Coburn (New York: Academic Press, 1981), p 323.
[2] AE Bender, *Nutrition and Dietetic Foods* (New York: Chemical Publishing Co., Inc.), p 202.
[3] GC Cotzias, *Proceedings of the First Annual Conference on Trace Substances in Environmental Health*, ed DD Hemphill (Columbia, Missouri: University of Missouri Press, 1967), pp 5-19.
[4] W Mertz, in *Environmental Geochemistry in Health and Disease* (Washington, D.C.: The Geological Society of America, Inc, 1971), pp 197-202.
[5] JP Carter et al, "Chromium (III) in Hypoglycemia and in Impaired Glucose Utilization in Kwashiorkor," *American Journal of Clinical Nutrition* 21 (1968):195-202.
[6] RA Anderson et al, "Chromium Supplementation of Human Subjects: Effects on Glucose, Insulin and Lipid Variables," *Metabolism* 32 (1983):894-9.
[7] LH Stickland, *Biochemistry Journal* 44 (1949):190.
[8] E Chargaff and C Green, *Journal of Biology and Chemistry* 173 (1948):263.
[9] W Mertz, "Effects and Metabolism of Glucose Tolerance Factor," *Present Knowledge in Nutrition* 36 (1976):365-72.
[10] BL O'Dell, "Bioavailability of Trace Elements," *Nutrition Reviews* 42 (1984):301-8.
[11] WEC Wacker and BL Vallee, "Chromium, Manganese, Nickel, Iron and Other Metals in Ribonucleic Acid from Diverse Biological Sources," *Journal of Biology and Chemistry* 234 (1959):3257.
[12] W Mertz, "Chromium Occurrence and Function in Biological Systems," *Physiology Review* 49 (1969):163-239.
[13] PV Vittorio, EW Wright, and BE Sinnott, *Canadian Journal of Biochemistry and Biophysiology* 40 (1962):1677.
[14] IH Tipton, "Distribution of Trace Metals in the Human Body," in *Metal Binding in Medicine*, ed MJ Seven (Philadelphia: Lippincott, 1960), pp 27-42.
[15] V Maxia et al, "Selenium and Chromium Assay in Egyptian Foods and Blood of Egyptian Children by Activation Analysis," in *Nuclear Activation Techniques in the Life Sciences* 157 (1972):527-50.
[16] EG Offenbacher and FX Pi-Sunyer, "Temperature and pH Effects on the Release of Chromium from Stainless Steel into Water and Fruit Juices, *Journal of Agriculture and Food Chemistry* 31 (1983):89-92.
[17] RA Anderson and NA Bryden, "Concentration, Insulin Potentiation, and Absorption of Chromium in Beer," *Journal of Agriculture and Food Chemistry* 31 (1983):308-11.
[18] HA Schroeder, *The Trace Elements and Man: Some Positive and Negative Aspects* (Old Greenwich, Connecticut: Devin-Adair Company, 1973), p 120.
[19] RS Pekarek et al, *Federal Proceedings* 32 (1973):930.
[20] "Glucose Metabolism in Undernourished Pregnant Women," *Nutrition News* 8, published by the National Institute of Nutrition, Tarnaka, Hyderabad, 1987.
[21] IWF Davidson and RL Burt, "Physiologic Changes in Plasma Chromium of Normal and Pregnant Women: Effect of a Glucose Load," *American Journal of Obstetrics and Gynecology* 116 (1973):601.
[22] B Kamen and S Kamen, *Total Nutrition for Breast-Feeding Mothers* (Boston: Little, Brown and Company, 1986), p 118.
[23] CC Pfeiffer, *Zinc and Other Micro-Nutrients* (New Canaan, CT,: Keats Publ,, Inc., 1978), p 131.
[24] Personal interview with Gary Price Todd, M.D., Waynesville, North Carolina, May 7, 1990.
[25] CC Pfeiffer, *Mental and Elemental Nutrients: A Physician's Guide to Nutrition and Health Care* (New Canaan, Connecticut: Keats Publishing, Inc., 1975), p 131.
[26] Mertz et al, *Federal Proceedings* 33 (1974):2275.
[27] LH Storlien et al, "Effects of Sucrose Vs. Starch Diets on In Vivo Insulin Action, Thermogenesis, and Obesity in Rats," *American Journal of Clinical Nutrition* 47 (1988):421.
[28] WW Campbell et al, "Exercise Training and Dietary Chromium Effects on Glycogen, Glycogen Synthase, Phosphorylase and Total Protein in Rats," *Journal of Nutrition* 119 (1989):653-60.
[29] R Anderson et al, "Effects of Supplemental Chromium on Patients with Symptoms of Reactive Hypoglycemia," *Metabolism* 36 (1987):351-5.
[30] JS Borel and RA Anderson, "Chromium," in *Biochemistry of the Essential Ultratrace Elements*, ed E Frieden (New York: Plenum Press, 1984), pp 175-99.
[31] R Anderson et al, "Chromium Supplementation of Human Subjects: Effects on Glucose, Insulin, and Lipid Variables," *Metabolism* 32 (1983):894-9.
[32] JS Borel and RA Anderson, "Chromium," in *Biochemistry of the Essential Ultratrace Elements*, ed E Frieden, (New York: Plenum Press, 1984), pp 175-99.
[33] W Niedermeier and JH Griggs, "Trace Metal Composition of Synovial Fluid and Blood Serum of Patients with Rheumatoid Arthritis," *Journal of Chronic Diseases* 23 (1971):527-36.
[34] WW Campbell et al, "Exercise Training and Dietary Chromium Effects on Glycogen, Glycogen Synthase, Phosphorylase and Total Protein in Rats," *Journal of Nutrition* 119 (1989):653-60.
[35] CC Pfeiffer, *Zinc and Other Micro-Nutrients* (New Canaan, Ct,: Keats Publ, Inc., 1978), p 131.
[36] RA Duce, GL Hoffman, and WH Zoller, *Science* 187 (1975):59-61.

[37] S Langard, "Chromium," in *Metals in the Environment*, ed HA Waldron (New York: Academic Press, 1980), p 112.
[38] R Anderson and A Kozlovsky, "Chromium Intake, Absorption and Excretion of Subjects Consuming Self-Selected Diets," *American Journal of Clinical Nutrition* 41 (1985):1177-83.
[39] W Mertz and EE Roginski, "Chromium Metabolism: The Glucose Tolerance Factor," in *Newer Trace Elements in Nutrition*, eds Mertz and Cornatzer (New York: Marcel Dekker, 1971), pp 123-50.
[40] WH Allaway, *Advances in Agronomics* 20 (1968):235-74.
[41] JS Borel and RA Anderson, *Biochemistry of Essential Trace Minerals*, ed E Frieden (New York: Plenum Publishing Corp, 1984).
[42] SR Tannenbaum, "Vitamins and Minerals," in *Principles of Food Science*, part I: Food Chemistry, ed OR Fennema (New York: Marcel Dekker, Inc., 1976), p 351.
[43] J Kumpulainen et al, *Journal of Agricultural and Food Chemistry* 27 (1979):490.
[44] WW Campbell and RA Anderson, "Effects of Aerobic Exercise and Training on the Trace Minerals Chromium, Zinc and Copper," *Sports Medicine* 4 (1987):9-18.
[45] A Kozlovsky et al, "Effects of Diets High in Simple Sugars on Urinary Chromium Losses," *Metabolism* 35 (1986):515-18.
[46] R Masironi, WR Wolf, and W Mertz, "Chromium in Refined and Unrefined Sugars: Possible Nutritional Implications in the Etiology of Cardiovascular Diseases," *Bulletin of the World Health Organization* 49 (1973):322-4.
[47] Personal interview with Gary Price Todd, M.D., Waynesville, North Carolina, May 7, 1990.
[48] L Mervyn, *Minerals and Your Health* (New Canaan, Connecticut: Keats Publishing, Inc, 1981), p 17.
[49] HA Schroeder, *The Trace Elements and Man: Some Positive and Negative Aspects* (Old Greenwich, Connecticut: Devin-Adair Company, 1973), p 27.
[50] HA Schroeder, *The Trace Elements and Man: Some Positive and Negative Aspects* (Old Greenwich, Connecticut: Devin-Adair Company, 1973), p 128.
[51] HA Schroeder, "The Role of Chromium in Mammalian Nutrition," *American Journal of Clinical Nutrition* 21 (1968):230-44.
[52] RR Weiler and VK Chawla, in "Proceedings of the 12th Conference on Great Lakes Research," pp 801-8.
[53] LP Coyle, *The World Encyclopedia of Food* (New York: Facts on File, Inc., 1982), p. 367.
[54] B Kamen, *Cholesterol: New Facts, New Solutions* (Novato, California: Nutrition Encounter, 1990).
[55] HA Schroeder, *The Trace Elements and Man: Some Positive and Negative Aspects* (Old Greenwich, Connecticut: Devin-Adair Company, 1973), p 132.
[56] CC Pfeiffer, *Mental and Elemental Nutrients: A Physician's Guide to Nutrition and Health Care* (New Canaan, Connecticut: Keats Publishing, Inc., 1975), p 26.
[57] HA Schroeder, *The Trace Elements and Man: Some Positive and Negative Aspects* (Old Greenwich, Connecticut: Devin-Adair Company, 1973), p 126.
[58] H Kather and B Simon, "Opioid Peptides and Obesity," *Lancet* 2 (1979):905.
[59] CC Pfeiffer, *Zinc and Other Micro-Nutrients* (New Canaan, Ct: Keats Publ, Inc. 1978), p 127.
[60] A Kramer, *Food and the Consumer* (Westport, CT, AVI Publishing Company, Inc., 1973), p 143.
[61] RS Harris and E Karmas, "*Nutritional Evaluation of food Processing* (Westport, Connecticut: The AVI Publishing Co., Inc, 1975), p 345.
[62] BT Hunter, *Food Additives and Federal Policy: The Mirage of Safety* (New York: Charles Scribner's Sons, 1975), p 35.
[63] "Diabetes: Nutritional Factors." Lecture presented by GP Todd, MD, Waynesville, North Carolina, in 1988.
[64] B Kamen, *Total Nutrition for Breast-Feeding Mothers,* (Boston: Little, Brown & Co, 1986), p 9.
[65] E Boyle, Jr., B Mondschein, and HH Dash, "Chromium Depletion in the Pathogenesis of Diabetes and Atherosclerosis," *Southern Medical Journal* 70 (1977):14549-53.
[66] T Noreth, "The Carcinogenicity of Chromium," *Environmental Health Perspective* (1981):121-30.
[67] Dr. Ben Lane, personal interview, June 9, 1990.
[68] EW Toepfer, et al, "Chromium in Foods in Relation to Biological Activity," *Journal of Agriculture and Food Chemistry* 21 (1973):69-73.
[69] Hoppe-Seyler and Thierfelder, *Handbuch Der Physiologische-Und Pathologische-Chemischen Analyse* (New York: Springer-Verlag, 1955), p 1213.

REFERENCES: CHAPTER 2

EM Widdowson, "Nutritional Individuality," *Proceedings of the Nutrition Society* 21 (1962):121.
[2] AL Lehninger, *Short Course in Biochemistry* (New York: Worth Publishers, Inc., 1973), p 349.
[3] K Bergstrom et al, "Diet, Muscle Glycogen and Physical Performance," *Acta Physiology Scandinavica* 71 (1967):71.
[4] R Bannister, "Special Presentation: Health, Fitness, and Sport," *American Journal of Clinical Nutrition* 49 (1989):927-30.

[5] L Jorfeldt and J Wahren, "Human Forearm Muscle Metabolism During Exercise: Quantitative Aspects of Glucose Uptake and Lactate Production During Prolonged Exercise," *Clinical Science* 41 (1970):459-73.
[6] B Saltin, Experiment cited by PO Astrand and K Rodahl, in *Textbook of Work Physiology* (New York: McGraw Hill, 1970), p 466.
[7] C Foster, DL Costill, and WJ Fink, "Effect of Pre-Exercise Feeding on Endurance Performance," *Medical Science Sports* 11 (1979):1-5.
[8] D Massicotte et al, "Metabolic Response to (^{13}C) Glucose and (^{13}) Fructose Ingestion During Exercise," *Journal of Applied Physiology* 61 (1986):1180-4.
[9] H Guthrie, *Journal of Nutrition Education* 13 (1981):46.
[10] A Leaf and KB Frisa, "Eating for Health of for Athletic Performance?" *American Journal of Clinical Nutrition*, suppl 49 (1989):1066-9.
[11] EH Christensen and O Hansen, "Arbeitsfahigkeit und Ehrnahrung," *Scandinavia Archives of Physiology* 81 (1939):160-75.
[12] LJ Bogert, GM Briggs, DH Calloway, *Nutrition and Physical Fitness* (Philadelphia: WB Saunders Company, 1966), p 94-5.
[13] J Bergstrom, E Hultman, and AE Roch-Norlund, "Lactic Acid Accumulation in Connection with Fructose Infusion," *Acta Medical Scandinavia* 184 (1968):359.
[14] R Shephard, "Energy Balance in Humans," *Physiology and Biochemistry of Exercise* (New York: Praeger Publishers, 1982), p 8.
[15] LH Nilsson and E Hultman, "Liver and Muscle Glycogen in Man After Glucose and Fructose Infusion," *Scandinavian Journal of Clinical Laboratory Investigation* 32 (1973):325.
[16] JD Brooke, GJ Davies, and LF Green, "The Effects of Normal and Glucose Syrup Work Diets on the Performance of Racing Cyclists," *Journal of Sports and Medical Physical Fitness* 15 (1975):257-65.
J Karlsson and B Saltin, "Diet, Muscle Glycogen and Endurance Performance," *Journal of Applied Physilogy* 31 (1971):203-6.
[18] LF Green and R Bagley, "Ingestion of a Glucose Syrup Drink During Long Distance Canoeing," *British Journal of Sports Medicine* 6 (1972):125-8.
[19] DS Muckle, "Glucose Syrup Ingestion and Team Performance in Soccer," *British Journal of Sports Medicine* (1973):340-3.
[20] J Bergstrom et al, "Diet, Muscle Glycogen and Physical Performance," *Acta Physiologica Scandinavica* 71 (1967):140-50.
[21] V Niinimaa et al, "Characteristics of the Successful Dinghy Sailor," *Journal of Sports Medicine and Physical Fitness* 17 (1977):83-96.
[22] JD Brooke, "Effect of Initial Exercise on Blood Glucose," *Canadian Journal of Applied Sport Science* 3 (1978):181.
[23] SA Levine and PM Kidd, *Antioxidant Adaptation: Its Role in Free Radical Pathology* (San Leandro, CA: Biocurrents Division, Allergy Research Group, 1985).
[24] A Leaf, "What Constitutes Good Nutrition for the Athlete and Postathlete," *American Journal of Clinical Nutrition* 49 (1989):936-7.
[25] A Leaf, "What Constitutes Good Nutrition for the Athlete and Postathlete," *American Journal of Clinical Nutrition* 49 (1989):936-7.
[26] R Anderson, "Effect of Exercise (Running) on Serum Glucose, Insulin, Glucagon, and Chromium Excretion," *Diabetes* 31 (1982):212-16.
[27] WW Campbell and RA Anderson, "Effects of Aerobic Exercise and Training on the Trace Minerals Chromium, Zinc and Copper," *Sports Medicine* 4 (1987):9-18.
[28] R Shephard, "Energy Balance in Humans," *Physiology and Biochemistry of Exercise* (New York: Praeger Publishers, 1982), p 13.
[29] D Donaldson et al, "Renal Excretion of Orally and Parenterally Administered Chromium-51," *Federal Proceedings* 41 (1982):391.
[30] W Campbell and R Anderson, "Effects of Aerobic Exercise and Training on the Trace Mineral Chromium, Zinc and Copper," *Sports Medicine* 4 (1987):9-18.
[31] EA Newsholme and AR Leech, *Biochemistry for Medical Sciences* (New York: Wiley, 1983).
[32] RW Rosebrough and NC Steele, "Effect of Supplemental Dietary Chromium or Nicotinic Acid on Carbohydrate Metabolism During Basal, Starvation, and Refeeding Periods in Poults," *Poultry Science* 60 (1981):407-17.
[33] G Saner, *Current Topics in Nutrition and Disease, vol 2: Chromium in Nutrition and Disease* (New York: Alan R Liss, Inc, 1980), p 12.
[34] CD Seaborn and BJ Stoecker, "Effects of Starch, Sucrose, Fructose and Glucose on Chromium Absorption and Tissue Concentrations in Obese and Lean Mice," *Journal of Nutrition* 10 (1989):1444-51.

REFERENCES: CHAPTER 3

[1] Personal interview, Gary Price Todd, M.D., Waynesville, North Carolina, May 7, 1990.
[2] Hippocrates, circa 410 BC.
[3] L Prokop, "International Olympic Committee Medical Commission's Policies and Programs in Nutrition and Physical Fitness," *American Journal of Clinical Nutrition,* suppl 49 (1989):1065.
[4] JR Brotherhood, "Nutrition and Sports Performance," *Sports Medicine* (1984):350-89.
[5] EA Richter, T Ploug, and H Galbo, "Increased Muscle Glucose Uptake After Exercise," *Diabetes* 34 (1985):1041-8.
[6] LP Garetto, EA Richter, and NB Ruderman, "Enhanced Muscle Glucose Metabolism After Exercise In Rat: The Two Phases," *American Journal of Physiology* 246; *Endocrinology Metabolism* 9 (1984):E471-E475, 1984.
[7] B Dufaux, G Assmann, and W Hollman, "Plasma Lipoproteins and Physical Activity: A Review," *International Journal of Sports Medicine* 3 (1982):123-36.
[8] RA Anderson et al, "Exercise Effects on Chromium Excretion of Trained and Untrained Men Consuming a Constant Diet," *Journal of Applied Physiology* 64 (1988):249-52.
[9] AL Lehninger, *Short Course in Biochemistry* (New York: Worth Publishers, Inc., 1973), p 162.
[10] ES Horton, "Metabolic Fuels, Utilization, and Exercise, "*American Journal Of Clinical Nutrition*, suppl 49 (1989):931-2.
[11] RA Anderson et al, "Exercise Effects on Chromium Excretion of Trained and Untrained Men Consuming a Constant Diet," *Journal of Applied Physiology* 64 (1988):249-52.
[12] V Koivisto et al, "Influence of Physical Training on the Fuel-Hormone Response to Prolonged Low Intensity Exercise," *Metabolism* 31 (1982):192-7.
[13] PD Gollnick and B Saltin, "Significance of Skeletal Muscle Oxidative Enzyme Enhancement with Endurance Training," *Clinical Physiology* 2 (1982):1-12.
[14] JD Chen, "Nutritional Problems and Measures in Elite and Amateur Athletes," *American Journal of Clinical Nutrition* suppl 49 (1989):1084-9.
[15] JD Chen, "Nutritional Problems and Measures in Elite and Amateur Athletes," *American Journal of Clinical Nutrition* suppl 49 (1989):1084-9.
[16] L Jorfeldt and J Wahren, "Human Forearm Muscle Metabolism During Exercise," V Quantitative Aspects of Glucose Uptake and Lactate Production During Prolonged Exercise, *Scandinavian Journal of Clinical Laboratory Investigation* 26 (1970):71-81.
[17] R Bannister, Special presentation, "Health, Fitness, and Sport," *American Journal Of Clinical Nutrition*, suppl 49 (1989):927-30.
[18] Physician's Desk Reference.
[19] Ibid.
[20] W Mertz et al, *Federal Proceedings* 23 (1974):2275.
[21] JS Borel and RA Anderson, "Chromium," in *Biochemistry of the Essential Ultratrace Elements,* ed E Frieden (New York: Plenum Press, 1984), pp 175-99.
[22] A Guyton, *Textbook of Medical Physiology* 7th ed (Phil:: WB Saunders Co, 1986), pp 923-30.
[23] GM Reaven, "Mono- and Disaccharide Metabolism in Feasting and Fasting," in *Carbohydrates and Health,* eds LF Hood et al (Westport, Connecticut: AVI Publishing Co, Inc, 1977), p 19.
[24] AR Loosli, "Athletes, Food and Nutrition," *Food and Nutrition News* 62, publication of the National Live Stock and Meat Board Research Department (1990):15-18.
[25] AC Grandjean, "Macronutrient Intake of US Athletes Compared with the General Population and Recommendations Made for Athletes," *American Journal of Clinical Nutrition,* suppl 49 (1989):1070.-5.
[26] JL Ivy et al, "Muscle Glycogen Synthesis After Exercise: Effect of Time of Carbohydrate Ingestion," *Journal of Applied Physiology* 64 (1988):1480-5.
[27] G Evans et al, "Interaction of the Glucose Tolerance Factor (GTF) with Insulin," *Chromium in Biological Systems, Biochemistry and Biophysical Research Committee* 50 (1973):718-22.
[28] B Saltin and L Hermansen, "Glycogen Stores and Prolonged Severe Exercise," in *Nutrition and Physical Activity,* ed G Blix, (Uppsala: Almqvist & Wiksell, 1967), p 32.
[29] Shepard, *Exercise*, p. 294.
[30] Guyton, op cit.
[31] HS Mitchell et al, *Nutrition in Health and Disease* 17th ed (Philadelphia: JB Lippincott Company, 1982), p. 153.
[32] R DeFronzo, "Insulin Secretion, Insulin Resistance and Obesity," *International Journal of Obesity* 6, Suppl 1 (1982):73-82.
[33] M Centanni et al, "Insulin Effect on Thyroid Hormone Uptake in Rat Skeletal Muscle," *Metabolism* 7 (1988):626-30.
[34] F Strand, *Physiology: A Regulatory Systems Approach,* 2nd ed 19 (New York: MacMillan Publishing company, 1983), p. 353.
[35] Ibid.

[36] VR Young, "Protein and Amino Acid Metabolism in Relation to Physical Exercise," in *Current Concepts in Nutrition*, vol 15, ed M Winick (New York: John Wiley & Sons, 1986), pp 9-32.
[37] E Hultman, "Nutritional Effects on Work Performance," *American Journal of Clinical Nutrition* 49 (1989):949-57.
[38] B Kamen, *Startling New Facts About Osteoporosis* (Novato, California: Nutrition Encounter, 1989).
[39] JD Chen, "Nutritional Problems and Measures in Elite and Amateur Athletes," *American Journal of Clinical Nutrition* suppl 49 (1989):1084-89.
[40] AR Loosli, "Athletes, Food and Nutrition," *Food and Nutrition News* 62, publication of the National Live Stock and Meat Board Research Department (1990):15-18.
[41] PWR Lemon, KE Yarasheski, and DG Dolny, "The Importance of Protein for Athletes," *Sports Medicine* 1 (1984):124-33.
[42] R Bannister, Special presentation, "Health, Fitness, and Sport," *American Journal Of Clinical Nutrition*, suppl 49 (1989):929.
[43] R Shephard, "Effects of Age and Sex Upon Energy Exchange," *Physiology and Biochemistry of Exercise* (New York: Praeger Publishers, 1982), p 323.
[44] C Williams, "Diet and Endurance Fitness," *American Journal of Clinical Nutrition* 49 (1989):1077-83.
[45] PO Astrand, "Diet and Athletic Performance," *Federal Proceedings* 26 (1967):1772-7.
[46] World Health Organization, "Expert Group in Requirements of Vitamin A, Thiamine, Riboflavin, and Niacin," *WHO Technical Report*, Series No. 362.
[47] E Hultman, "Nutritional Effects on Work Performance," *American Journal of Clinical Nutrition*, suppl 49 (1989):949-57.
[48] Shephard, "Limitations Upon the Rate of Working," *Exercise*, p 85.
[49] RM Restak, *The Mind* (New York: Bantam Books, 1988), p 75.
[50] L Prokop, "International Olympic Committee Medical Commission's Policies and Programs in Nutrition and Physical Fitness," *American Journal of Clinical Nutrition*, suppl 49 (1989):1065.

REFERENCES: CHAPTER 4

[1] RM Restak, *The Mind* (New York: Bantam Books, 1988), p 75.
[2] WR Harlan et al, "Secular Trends in Body Mass in the United States, 1960-1980" *American Journal of Epidemiology* 128 (1988):1065-74.
[3] National Institutes of Health Consensus Development Panel on the Health Implications of Obesity. Health Implications of Obesity: National Institutes of Health Consensus Development Conference Statement. *Annals of Internal Medicine* 103 (1985):1073-7.
[4] TB Van Itllie, "Obesity: Adverse Effects on Health and Longevity, *American Journal of Clinical Nutrition* suppl 32 (1979):2723-33.
[5] EL Bierman and J Hirsch, in *Textbook of Endocrinology*, ed RH Williams (Philadelphia: WB Saunders, 1981), 907-21.
[6] GV Mann, "The Influence of Obesity on Health," *New England Journal of Medicine* 291 (1974):178-85,226-32.
[7] E Cheraskin, WM Ringsdorf, Jr., and A Brecher, *Psychodietetics* (NY: Stein and Day, 1974), p. 36.
[8] KD Brownell, "Weight Cycling," *American Journal of Clinical Nutrition* suppl 49 (1989):937.
[9] PA Kern et al, "The Effects of Weight Loss on the Activity and Expression of Adipose-Tissue Lipoprotein Lipase in Very Obese Humans," *New England Journal of Medicine* 322 (1990):1053-9.
[10] T Cox, *Stress* (Baltimore: University Park Press, 1978), p 69.
[11] S Woods et al, "Insulin: Its Relationship to the Central Nervous System and to the Control of Food Intake and Body Weight," *American Journal of Clinical Nutrition* 42 (1985):1063-71.
[12] D Weatherall et al, *Oxford Textbook of Medicine* (Oxford, England: Oxford University Press, 1987), p 64.
[13] S Zuniga-Guarjdo et al, "Effects of Obesity on Insulin Sensitivity and Insulin Clearance and the Metabolic Response to Insulin as Assessed by the Euglycemic Insulin Clamp Technique," *Metabolism* 35 (1986):278-82.
[14] P Bondy and L Rosenberg, *Metabolic Control and Disease*, 8th ed (Philadelphia: WB Saunders Company, 1989), p. 509.
[15] D Foster, "Insulin Resistance: A Secret Killer?" *New England Journal of Medicine* 11 (1989):733-4.
[6] Bondy, op cit.
[17] A Guyton, *Textbook of Medical Physiology* 5th ed (Phil: WB Saunders Company, 1976), p 973.
[18] J Mayer, "Genetic, Traumatic and Environmental Factors in the Etiology of Obesity," *Physicians Review* 33 (1953):472-508.
[19] A Debons, "Rapid Effects of Insulin on the Hypothalamic Satiety Center," *American Journal of Physiology* 216 (1969):1114-18.
[20] M Van Houton and B Posner, "Cellular Basis of Direct Insulin Action in the Central Nervous System," *Diabetologia* 20 (1981):255-67.
[21] D Porte and S Woods, "Regulation of Food Intake and Body Weight by Insulin," *Diabetologia* 20 (1981):274-80.

[22] S Woods et al, "Insulin: Its Relationship to the Central Nervous System and to the Control of Food Intake and Body Weight," *American Journal of Clinical Nutrition* 42 (1985):1063-71.
[23] M Virkkunen and S Narvanan, "Plasma Insulin, Tryptophan and Serotonin Levels During the Glucose Tolerance Test Among Habitually Violent and Impulsive Offenders," *Neuropsychobiology* 17 (1987):19-23.
[24] P Roland and V Augusto, "Facilitating Effect of Insulin on Brain 5-Hydroxytryptamine Metabolism," *Neuroendocrinology* 45 (1987):267-273.
[25] R Wurtman and J Wurtman, "Carbohydrate Craving, Obesity and Brain Serotonin," *Appetite* 7 (1986):99-103.
[26] B Caballero, "Insulin Resistance and Amino Acid Metabolism in Obesity," *New York Academy of Science Annals* 499 (1987):84-93.
[27] D Ashley et al, "Evidence for Diminished Brain 5-Hydroxytryptamine Biosynthesis in Obese Diabetic and Non-Diabetic Humans," *American Journal of Clinical Nutrition* 42 (1985):1240-45.
[28] A Tremblay, "Impact of Dietary Fat Content and Fat Oxidation on Energy Intake in Humans," *American Journal of Clinical Nutrition* 49 (1989):799-805.
[29] Personal interview with George Boucher, April 1990. Unpublished.
[30] R Riales and MJ Albrink, "Effect of Chromium Chloride Supplementation on Glucose Tolerance and Serum Lipids Including High-Density Lipoprotein of Adult Men," *American Journal of Clinical Nutrition* 34 (1981):2670-8.
[31] FA Jeannet and B Jeanrenaud, "The Hormonal and Metabolic Basis of Experimental Obesity," *Clinical Endocrinology and Metabolism* 5 (1976):337-66.
[32] H Freund et al, "Chromium Deficiency During Total Parenteral Nutrition," *Journal of the American Medical Association* 241 (1981):496-8.
[33] M McCarty, "Chromium and Insulin," *American Journal of Clinical Nutrition* 36 (1982):384.
[34] DA Thompson and RG Campbell, "Hunger in Man Induced by 2-Deoxy-D-Glucose: Glucoprivic Control of Taste Preference of Food Intake," *Science* 198 (1977):1065-8.
[35] J Wurtman et al, "Impaired Control of Appetite for Carbohydrates in Some Patients with Eating Disorders: Treatment with Pharmacological Agents," in *Psychobiology of Anorexia Nervosa* (New York: Springer-Verlag, 1984), 12-21.
[36] J Wurtman and R Wurtman, "Drugs that Enhance Central Serotoninergic Transmission Diminish Elective Carbohydrate Consumption by Rats," *Life Sciences* 24 (1979):895-904.
[37] A Guyton, *Textbook of Medical Physiology*, 5th ed (Phil: WB Saunders Company, 1976), p 923.
[38] R Cavalieri and R Basil, "Impaired Peripheral Conversion of Thyroxine to Triidothyronine," *Annals of Review of Medicine* 28 (1977):57-65.
[39] M Centanni et al, "Insulin Effect on Thyroid Hormone Uptake in Rat Skeletal Muscle," *Metabolism* 37 (1988):626-30.
[40] R Roxen et al, "Effects of 'Physiological' Dose of Triidothyronine on Obese Subjects During a Protein-Sparing Diet," *International Journal of Obesity* 10 (1986):303-12.
[41] R DeFronzo, "Insulin Secretion, Insulin Resistance and Obesity," *International Journal of Obesity* 6, Suppl 1 (1982):73-82.
[42] GB Haber, KW Heaton, and D Murphy, "Depletion and Disruption of Dietary Fiber," *Lancet* 2 (1977):679-82.
[43] M Modan et al, "Effect of Diet, Past and Recent, and Energy Expenditures in Daily Living Activities on Rate of Glucose Intolerance: The Israel GOH Study," Poster presentation, First International Conference on Nutrition and Fitness, 1988, reported in *American Journal Of Clinical Nutrition* suppl 49 (1989):1133-4.
[44] MF McCarty, "Chromium and Insulin," *American Journal of Clinical Nutrition* 36 (1982):384.
[45] WPT James, "The Role of Nutrition and Fitness in Chronic Diseases," *American Journal Of Clinical Nutrition* suppl 49 (1989):931-2.

REFERENCES: CHAPTER 5

[1] H Selye, *The Stress of Life* (New York: McGraw-Hill Book Company, 1976).
[2] M Ermini, "Aging As A Biological Process: A Perspective," in *Aging, Immunity and Arthritis Disease*, vol 2, eds MB Kay et al (New York: Raven Press, 1980), p 8.
[3] T Cox, *Stress* (Baltimore: University Park Press, 1978), p 56.
[4] JW Mason, "Organization of Psychoendocrine Mechanisms," *Psychosomatic Medicine* 30, part 2 (1968).
[5] JW Mason, "Emotion as Reflected in Patterns of Endocrine Integration," in *Emotions: Their Parameters and Measurement*, ed L Levi (New York: Raven Press, 1975).
[6] TA Rennie and JE Howard, "Hypoglycemia and Tension Depression," *Psychosomatic Medicine* 4 (1942):273.
[7] J Biermann and B Toohey, *The Diabetic's Book* (Los Angeles: JP Tarcher, Inc, 1981).
[8] JH Growdon, "Neurotransmitter Precursors in the Diet: Their Use in the Treatment of Brain Diseases," in *Nutrition and the Brain*, vol 3, eds JR Wurtman and JJ Wurtman (New York: Raven Press, 1979), p 125.
[9] RS Lazarus, *Patterns of Adjustment* (New York: McGraw-Hill, 1966).

[10] T Cox, GC Simpson, and DR Rothschild, "Blood Glucose Level and Skilled Performance Under Stress," *Journal of International Research Communications* 1 (1973):30.
[11] JD Brooke et al, "Dietary Pattern of Carbohydrate Provision and Accident Incidence in Foundry Men," *Proceedings of the Nutrition Society* 32 (1973):44.
[12] JD Brooke et al, "Factory Accidents and Carbohydrate Supplements," *Proceedings of the Nutrition Society* 32 (1973):94.
[13] P Slagle, *The Way Up from Down* (New York: Random House, 1987), p 95.
[14] J Froberg et al, "Physiological and Biochemical Stress Reactions Induced by Psychosocial Stimuli," in *Society, Stress and Disease*, vol 1, ed L Levi (New York: Oxford University Press, 1971).
[15] CC Pfeiffer, *Mental and Elemental Nutrients: A Physician's Guide to Nutrition and Health Care* (New Canaan, Connecticut: Keats Publishing, Inc., 1975), p 10.
[16] B Kamen, "The Stress Effect," *Let's Live Magazine*, October 1988.

REFERENCES: CHAPTER 6

[1] GM Reaven, Banting Lecture 1988, "Role of Insulin Resistance in Human Disease," *Diabetes* 37 (1988):1595-607
[2] GD Calvert et al, "Effects of Therapy on Plasma-High-Density-Lipo-Protein-Cholesterol Concentration in Diabetes Mellitus," *Lancet* 2 (1978):66-8.
[3] M Simonoff, "Chromium Deficiency and Cardiovascular Risk," *Cardiovascular Research* 18 (1984):591-6.
[4] I Zavaroni et al, 'Risk Factors for Coronary Artery Disease in Healthy Persons with Hyperinsulinemia and Normal Glucose Tolerance," *New England Journal of Medicine* 320 (1989):702-6.
[5] ME Rosenbaum, MD, "Nutrition Watch," KNBC radio interview with Betty Kamen, May 1989.
[6] M Chen, RN Bergman, and D Porte, Jr., "Insulin Resistance and B-Cell Dysfunction in Aging: The Importance of Dietary Carbohydrate," *Journal of Clinical Endocrinology and Metabolism* 67 (1988):951-7.
[7] T Gordon et al, "High Density Lipoprotein as a Protective Factor Against Coronary Heart Disease," The Framingham Study, *American Journal of Medicine* 62 (1977):707.
[8] N Miller et al, "The Tromso Heart-Study High-Density Lipoprotein and Coronary Heart Disease: A Prospective Case Control Study," *Lancet* 1 (1977):965.
[9] G Rhoads et al, "Serum Lipoproteins and Coronary Heart Disease in a Population Study of Hawaii Japanese Men," *New England Journal of Medicine* 294 (1976):293.
[10] A Walker and B Walker, "High High-Density Lipoprotein Cholesterol in African Children and Adults in a Population Free of Coronary Heart Disease," *British Medical Journal* 2 (1978):1336-7.
[11] D Burkitt and H Trowell, *Refined Carbohydrate Foods and Disease* (London: Academic Press, 1975).
[12] HA Schroeder, "The Role of Chromium in Mammalian Nutrition," *American Journal of Clinical Nutrition* 21 (1968):230-44.
[13] H Schroeder and J Balassa, "Influence of Chromium, Cadmium, and Lead in Rat Aortic Lipids and Circulating Cholesterol," *American Journal of Physiology* 209 (1965):433-7.
[14] D Nash et al, "The Effect of Brewer's Yeast Containing Rich Glucose Tolerance Factor on Serum Lipids," *Proceedings of the 5th International Symposium on Atherosclerosis*, Houston, Texas, 1979.
[15] EG Offenbacher and X Pi-Sunyer, "Effect of Chromium-Rich Yeast on Glucose Tolerance and Blood Lipids in Elderly Subjects," *Diabetes* 29 (1980):919-25.
[16] A Abraham et al, "The Effects of Chromium on Established Atherosclerotic Plaques in Rabbits," *American Journal of Clinical Nutrition* 33 (1980):2294-8.
[17] H Schroeder et al, "Chromium Deficiency as a Factor in Atherosclerosis," *Journal of Chronic Diseases* 23 (1970):123-42.
[18] H Newman et al, "Serum Chromium and Angiographically Determined Coronary Artery Disease," *Clinical Chemistry* 24 (1978):541-4.
[19] R Riales and MJ Albrink, "Effect of Chromium Chloride Supplementation on Glucose Tolerance and Serum Lipids Including High-Density Lipoproteins of Adult Men," *American Journal of Clinical Nutrition* 34 (1981):2670-8.
[20] R Riales and MJ Albrink, "Effect of Chromium Chloride Supplementation on Glucose Tolerance and Serum Lipids Including High-Density Lipoproteins of Adult Men," *American Journal of Clinical Nutrition* 34 (1981):2670-8.
[21] HA Schroeder, "The Role of Chromium in Mammalian Nutrition," *American Journal of Clinical Nutrition* 21 (1968):230-44.
[22] HW Staub, G Reussner, and R Thiessen, Jr, "Serum Cholesterol Reduction by Chromium in Hypercholesterolemic Rats," *Science* 166 (1969):746.
[23] RL Patten et al, "Association of Plasma High-Density Lipoprotein Cholesterol with Clinical Chemistry Data," Lipid Research Clinics Program Prevalence Study, *Circulation* 62, suppl IV (1980):62.
[24] Council on Scientific Affairs, "Dietary and Pharmacologic Therapy for the Lipid Risk Factors," *Journal of the American Medical Association* 250 (1983):1873-9.
[25] "Best-Selling Cholesterol Book Sparks $6-Million Lawsuit," *Ann Arbor News*, December 12, 1988.

[26] MR Goldstein, "Potential Problems with the Widespread Use of Niacin," *American Journal of Medicine* 85 (1988):881.
[27] GE Mullin et al, "Fulminant Hepatic Failure After Ingestion of Sustained-Release Nicotinic Acid," *Annals of Internal Medicine* 111 (1989):253-5.
[28] MC Mitchell, Jr., Division of Gastroenterology, The Johns Hopkins School of Medicine, Baltimore. Interview, *Preventive Medicine Update*, November 1989.
[29] J Urberg, J Benyi, and R John, "Hypocholesterolemic
Effects of Nicotinic Acid and Chromium Supplementation," *Journal of Family Practice* 27 (1988):603-6.
[30] W Mertz, "Effects and Metabolism of the Glucose Tolerance Factor," *Present Knowledge in Nutrition* 36, Nutrition Foundation, Washington, DC, 1976, pp. 365-72.
[31] Interview with R Anderson, United States Department of Agriculture, KNBC radio, April 1989.
[32] JL Cutts and AD Bankhurst, "Suppression of Lymphoid Cell Function In Vitro by Inhibition of 3-Hydroxy-3-Methylglutaryl Coenzyme A Reductase by Lovastatin," *International Journal of Immunopharmacology* 11 (1989):863-9.
[33] HD Itskovitz et al, "Effect of Lovastatin on Serum Lipids in Patients With Nonfamilial Primary Hypercholesterolemia," *Clinical Therapy* 11 (1989):228-30.
[34] RS Paffenbarger and RT Hyde, "Exercise as a Protection Against Coronary Heart Disease," *New England Journal of Medicine* 302 (1980):726-1027.
[35] RK Peters et al, "Physical Fitness and Subsequent Myocardial Infarction in Healthy Workers, *Journal of the American Medical Association* 249 (1983):3052-6.
[36] JN Morris et al, "Vigorous Exercise in Leisure Time: Protection Against Coronary Heart Disease," *Lancet* 2 (1980):1207-10.
[37] M Simonoff, "Chromium Deficiency and Cardiovascular Risk," *Cardiovascular Research* 18 (1984):591-6.
[38] R Stout, "The Relationship of Abnormal Circulating Insulin Levels to Atherosclerosis," *Atherosclerosis* 27 (1977):1-13.
[39] K Pyorala, "Relationship of Glucose Tolerance and Plasma Insulin to the Incidence of Coronary Heart Disease: Results from Two Population Studies in Finland," *Diabetes Care* 2 (1975):131-41.
[40] J Mann and W Inman, "Oral Contraceptives and Death from Myocardial Infarction," *British Medical Journal* 2 (1975):245.
[41] P Back, "Contraceptive Steroids: Modification of Carbohydrate and Lipid Metabolism," *Metabolism* 22 (1973):841-55.
[42] WN Spellacy et al, "Glucose, Insulin and Growth Hormone Studies in Long-Term Users of Oral Contraceptives," *American Journal of Obstetrics and Gynecology* 106 (1970):173.
[43] HA Schroeder, "The Role of Chromium in Mammalian Nutrition," *American Journal of Clinical Nutrition* 21 (1968):230-44.
[44] HW Staub, G Reussner, and R Thiessen, Jr., "Serum Cholesterol Reduction by Chromium in Hyper-cholesterolemic Rats," *Science* 166 (1969):746.
[45] M Simonoff, "Chromium Deficiency and Cardiovascular Risk," *Cardiovascular Research* 18 (1984):591-6.

REFERENCES: CHAPTER 7

[1] CC Pfeiffer, *Zinc and Other Micro-Nutrients* (New Canaan, Connecticut: Keats Publishing, Inc., 1978), pp 126-33.
[2] G Saner, "Chromium Metabolism in Aged Subjects," *Current Topics in Nutrition and Disease, vol II: Chromium in Nutrition and Disease* (New York: Alan L Liss, 1980), p 117.
[3] DF Sims and EA Sims, *The "Other" Diabetes*, American Diabetes Association, 1982.
[4] "Chromium Protects Against Adult Onset Diabetes," News Release, Federation of American Societies for Experimental Biology, Office of Public Affairs, Bethesda, MD, April 3, 1990.
[5] W Mertz, "Effects and Metabolism of the Glucose Tolerance Factor," *Present Knowledge in Nutrition* 36, The Nutrition Foundation, Washington, DC, 1976.
[6] CR Kahn, "Role of Insulin Receptors in Insulin-Resistant States," *Metabolism* 29 (1980):455-66.
[7] KM Hambidge et al, "Concentration of Chromium in the Hair of Normal Children and Children with Juvenile Diabetes Mellitus," *Diabetes* 17 (1968):517.
[8] JM Morgan, "Hepatic Chromium Content in Diabetic Subjects," *Metabolism* 21 (1972):313.
[9] RJ Doisy et al, "Chromium Metabolism in Man in Trace Elements in Human Health and Disease, in *Nutrition Foundation Monograph*, ed AS Prasad (New York: Academic Press, 1976), p 79.
[10] DA Thompson, "Flameless Atomic Absorption Spectroscopy of Plasma Chromium," *American Clinical Biochemistry* 17 (1980):144.
[11] [[[august 10, 89 p. 370 - ref # 84.
[12] DW Foster, "Insulin Resistance: A Secret Killer?" *New England Journal of Medicine* 320 (1989):733-4.
[13] AF Casparie and LD Elving, "Severe Hypoglycemia in Diabetic Patients: Frequency, Causes, Prevention," *Diabetes Care* 8 (1985):134-40.
[14] E Glaser and G Halpern, *Biochemistry* 207 (1929):292.

[15] DR Hadden et al, "Maturity Onset Diabetes Mellitus: Response to Intensive Dietary Management, *British Medical Journal* 3 (1975):276-8.
[16] JL Leahy et al, "Chronic Hyperglycemia is Associated with Impaired Glucose Influence on Insulin Secretion: A Study of Normal Rats Using Chronic In Vivo Glucose Infusions," *Journal of Clinical Investigation* 77 (1986):908-15.
[17] RD Lawrence, "The Effect of Exercise on Insulin Action in Diabetics," *British Medical Journal* 1 (1926):648-50.
[18] J Wahren, L Hagenfeldt, and P Felig, "Splanchnic and Leg Exchange of Glucose, Amino Acids, and Free Fatty Acids During Exercise in Diabetes Mellitus," *Clinical Investigation* 55 (1975):1303-14.
[19] J Wahren et al, "Glucose Metabolism During Leg Exercise in Man," *Journal of Clinical Investigation* 50 (1971):15-25.
[20] J Erikson et al, "Early Metabolic Defects in Persons at Increased Risk for Non-Insulin-Dependent Diabetes Mellitus," *New England Journal of Medicine* 321 (1989):337-43.
[21] DR McCance, "Long-Term Glycemic Control and Diabetic Retinopathy," *Lancet* 2 (1989):824-7.
[22] KS Polonsky et al, "Abnormal Patterns of Insulin Secretion in Non-Insulin-Dependent Diabetes Mellitus," *New England Journal of Medicine* 318 (1988):1231-9.
[23] RW Stout, "The Relationship of Abnormal Circulating Insulin Levels to Atherosclerosis," *Atherosclerosis* 27 (1977):1-13.
[24] B Zinman, "The Physiologic Replacement of Insulin," *New England Journal of Medicine* 321 (1989):363-70.
[25] DC Robbins, EF Normand, and JP Colnes, *New England Journal of Medicine* 310 (1984):1388-9.
[26] DJ Jenkins, RH Taylor, and TMS Wolever, "The Diabetic Diet, Dietary Carbohydrate and Differences in Digestibility," *Diabetologia* 21 (1982):477-84.
[27] GP Todd, "Diabetes: Nutritional Factors," lecture presentation on tape, Waynesville, NC, 1988.
[28] RK Bernstein, *Diabetes: The Glucograf Method for Normalizing Blood Sugar* (New York: Crown Publishers, Inc., 1981), p 164.
[29] D Collings, G Williams, and I Macdonald, "Effects of Cooking on Serum Glucose and Insulin Responses to Starch," *British Medical Journal* 282 (1981):1032.
[30] AM Fontvieille et al, "A Moderate Switch from High to Low Glycemic-Index Foods for Three Weeks Improves Metabolic Control of Type I (IDDM) Diabetic Subjects," *Diabetes Nutrition Metabolism* 1 (1988):139-43.
[31] DJA Jenkins et al, "Exceptionally Low Blood Glucose Response to Dried Beans; Comparison With Other Carbohydrate Foods," *British Medical Journal* 2 (1980):578-80.
[32] "Glucose Metabolism in Undernourished Pregnant Women," *Nutrition News* 8, publication of the National Institute of Nutrition, Tarnaka, Hyderabad, India, 1987.
[33] *Lancet*
[34] LL Hopkins, Jr., O Ransome-Kuti, and AS Majaj, "Improvement of Impaired Carbohydrate Metabolism by Chromium (III) in Malnourished Infants," *American Journal of Clinical Nutrition* 21 (1968):531-4.
[35] H Schroeder, J Balassa, and I Tipton, "Abnormal Trace Metals in Man: Chromium," *Journal of Chronic Diseases* 15 (1962):941-64.
[36] Pfeiffer, *Micro-Nutrients*, op cit, p 127.
[37] A Burchell et al, "Hepatic Microsomal Glucose-6-Phophatase System and Sudden Infant Death Syndrome," *Lancet* 2 (1989):292-3.
[38] HA Schroeder, *The Trace Elements and Man* (Old Greenwich, Connecticut: Devin-Adair Company, 1973), p 64.
[39] RA Anderson et al, "Effects of Supplemental Chromium on Patients With Symptoms of Reactive Hypoglycemia," *Metabolism* 36 (1987):351-5.
[40] RA Anderson et al, "[[[]]]," *American Journal of Clinical Nutrition* 36 (1982):1184.
[41] RW Tuman, JT Bibo and RJ Doisy, "Comparison and Effects of Natural and Synthetic Glucose Tolerance Factor in Normal and Genetically Diabetic Mice," *Diabetes* 27 (1979):49.
[42] W Mertz, "Chromium Occurrence and Function in Biological Systems," *Physiology Reviews* 49 (1969):163.
[43] EE Roginski and W Mertz, "Effects Of Chromium (III) Supplementation On Glucose And Amino Acid Metabolism In Rats Fed A Low Protein Diet," *Journal of Nutrition* 97 (1969):525-30.
[44] *Journal of the American Medical Association*," (1982).
[45] GP Todd, *Nutrition, Health, and Disease* (Norfolk, Virginia: The Donning Company, 1987), p 172.

REFERENCES: CHAPTER 8

[1] RA Anderson, "Chromium," in Trace Minerals in Foods, ed K Smith (New York: Marcel Dekker, Inc., 1988), p 231.
[2] WPT James, "The Role of Nutrition and Fitness in Chronic Diseases," *American Journal of Clinical Nutrition*, suppl 49 (1989):934.
[3] E Wisker, A Maltz, and W Feldheim, "Metabolizable Energy of Diets Low or High in Dietary Fiber from Cereals When Eaten by Humans," *Journal of Nutrition* 118 (1988):945-52.
[4] JC Brand et al, "Plasma Glucose and Insulin Responses to Traditional Pima Indian Meals," *American Journal Of Clinical Nutrition* 51 (1990):416-20.

[5] MJ Thorne, LU Thompson, and DJA Jenkins, "Factors Affecting Starch Digestibility and the Glycemic Response with Special Reference to Legumes," *American Journal Of Clinical Nutrition* 38 (1983)481-8.
[6] O Hamberg, JJ Rumessen, and E Gudmand-Hoyer, "Blood Glucose Response to Pea Fiber: Comparisons with Sugar Beet Fiber and Wheat Bran," *American Journal of Clinical Nutrition* 50 (1989):324-8.
[7] FRJ Bornet et al, "Insulin and Glycemic Responses in Healthy Humans to Native Starches Processed in Different Ways: Correlation with In Vitro a-Amylase Hydrolysis[1-3]," *American Journal of Clinical Nutrition* 50 (1989):315-23.
[8] E Ferrannini et al, "Effect of Fatty Acids on Glucose Production and Utilization in Man," *Journal of Clinical Investigation* 72 (1983):1737-47.
[9] HA Schroeder, *The Trace Elements and Man* (Old Greewich, Connecticut: Devin-Adair Company, 1973), p 55.
[10] KNBR radio interview with Richard A Anderson, United States Department of Agriculture, June 18, 1989.
[11] J Bergstrom and E Hultman, *Journal of the American Medical Association* 221 (1972):999.
[12] W Mertz, "Chromium Occurrence and Function in Biological Systems," *Physiology Reviews* 49 (1969):163.
[13] CC Pfeiffer, *Mental and Elemental Nutrients: A Physician's Guide to Nutrition and Health Care* (New Canaan, Connecticut: Keats Publishing, Inc., 1975), p 293.
[14] IH Tipton and MJ Cooke, "Trace Elements in Human Tissue, Part 2: Adult Subjects from the United States," *Health Physiology* 9 (1963):103.
[15] IH Tipton et al, "Trace Elements in Human Tissue, Part 3: Subjects from Africa, The Near and Far East and Europe," *Health Physiology* 11 (1965):403.
16 RA Anderson, "Essentiality of Chromium in Humans," *Science of the Total Environment* 86 (1989):75-81.
[17] JA Cooper et al, "Structure and Biological Activity of Nitrogen and Oxygen Coordinated Nicotinic Acid Complexes of Chromium," *Inorganica Chimica Acta* 91, Elsevier Sequoia, Switzerland (1984):1-9.
[18] KM Hambidge, "Chromium," in *Disorders of Mineral Metabolism,* F Bronner and JW Coburn, eds, (New York: Academic Press, 1981), p 275.
[19] RA Anderson, "Nutritional Role of Chromium," *Science of the Total Environment* 17 (1981):13-29.
[20] M Simonoff, "Chromium Deficiency and Cardiovascular Risk," *Cardiovascular Research* 18 (1984):591-596.
[21] KM Hambidge, "Chromium," in *Disorders of Mineral Metabolism,* F Bronner and JW Coburn, eds, (New York: Academic Press, 1981), p 274.
[22] S Langard, "Chromium" in *Metals in the Environment* HA Waldron, ed (New York: Academic Press, 1980), p 112.
[23] W Mertz, "Chromium Occurrence and Function in Biological Systems," *Physiological Review* 49 (1969):163-239.
[24] R Anderson et al, "Effects of Chromium Supplementation on Urinary Chromium Excretion of Human Subjects and Correlation of Chromium Excretion with Selected Clinical Parameters," *Journal of Nutrition* 113 (1983):276-81.
[25] W Mertz et al, "Biological Activity and Fate of Trace Quantities of Intravenous Chromium (III) in the Rat," *American Journal of Physiology* 209 (1964):489-94.
[26] L Sherman et al, "Failure of Trivalent Chromium to Improve Hyperglycemia in Diabetes Mellitus," *Metabolism* 17 (1968):439.
[27] J Cooper et al, "Structure and Biological Activity of Nitrogen and Oxygen Coordinated Nicotinic Acid Complexes of Chromium," *Inorganica Chimica Acta* 91 (1984):1-9.
[28] RA Anderson, personal interview.
[29] *Archives of Environmental Health* 28 (1974).
[30] P Saltman, J Gurin, and I Mothner, *The California Nutrition Book* (New York: Little, Brown and Company, 1987), p 94.
[31] Schroeder, p. 132
[32] RA Levine et al, "Effect of Oral Chromium Supplementation on the Glucose Tolerance of Elderly Human Subjects," *Metabolism, Clinical Experiments* 17 (1968):114.
[33] LL Hopkins, Jr. and MG Price, "Effectiveness of Chromium (III) in Improving the Impaired Glucose Tolerance of Middle-Aged Americans, *Proceedings of the Western Hemisphere Nutritional Congress* 2nd, vol 2 (1968):40.
[34] RJ Doisy et al, "Chromium Metabolism in Man and Biochemical Effects," in *Trace Elements in Human Health and Disease,* vol 2, AS Prasad, ed (New York: Academic Press, 1976), pp. 79-104.
[35] R Shephard, "Energy Balance in Humans," *Physiology and Biochemistry of Exercise* (New York: Praeger Publishers, 1982), p 377.
[36] T Smith, *Exercise: Cult or Cure-All?* British Medical Journal 286 (1983):1637-9.
[37] A Leaf, "What Constitutes Good Nutrition for the Athlete and Postathlete," *American Journal of Clinical Nutrition* 49 (1989):936-7.

INDEX

NOTES

NOTES